To our families who have supported us in our work,
and to the many patients who have taught us
the lessons we impart to others.

Contents

Assessment Tools and Patient Resources   vi

Preface   vii

Acknowledgments   viii

Chapter 1   Introduction to Lifestyle Management   1

Chapter 2   Lifestyle Management: Theories of Intervention   7

Chapter 3   Education, Communication, and Methods
            of Intervention   21

Chapter 4   Psychological Issues Affecting Lifestyle Change   31

Chapter 5   Adherence to Exercise Programs   47

Chapter 6   Dietary Assessment and Intervention   61
            Mia Clark

Chapter 7   Stress Management   79

Chapter 8   Smoking Cessation   85

Chapter 9   Adherence to Medications   105

References   115

Index   127

About the Authors   133

Assessment Tools
and Patient Resources

Chapter 2   Hyperlipidemic Diet Intervention for MULTIFIT   19

Chapter 4   Psychosocial Questionnaire   38
            MULTIFIT Information for Spouses   40

Chapter 5   Pre-Exercise Assessment Questionnaire   55
            MULTIFIT Daily Exercise Log   56
            Weekly Exercise Activity Log   58
            Exercise Plan and Tip Sheet   59

Chapter 6   Sample Questions From the Food Frequency
                Questionnaire   73
            Food Frequency Assessment Tools   75
            Efficacy Questionnaire   76
            List of Cookbooks and Food Magazines   77
            CALS Dietary Intervention Components and Examples   78

Chapter 8   Physician Advice Statement for Smoking Cessation   95
            Fagerström Tolerance Test of Nicotine Dependence   96
            Nicotine Chewing Gum Patient Information   97
            Nicotine Transderm Patch (24 hour) Patient Information 99
            Self-Efficacy Questionnaire on Smoking   100
            Telephone Interview for Patients
                Attempting to Quit Smoking   101

Chapter 9   Medication Information Sheet   111

Preface

During the past decade there have been numerous advances in the care of patients with coronary heart disease. These changes—including both technological advances in treatment and a better understanding of the factors that influence the manifestation, pathogenesis, progression, and regression of coronary atherosclerosis—have led to an enhanced prognosis for many patients and an improvement in their quality of life. Over this period of time much has also been learned about efficacy of modifying coronary risk factors in this population, including the strategies needed to help patients maintain major lifestyle modifications. Such knowledge has led to a clearer understanding of the techniques health care professionals can employ to help patients in their process of change.

This monograph is designed to help all health care professionals who are involved in educating and counseling patients to modify coronary risk factors. We use a behavior-oriented approach to risk factor modification, drawing upon the more than 20 years of research and clinical experience of the Stanford Cardiac Rehabilitation Program. We provide a theoretical approach to risk factor modification, present methods for intervention, and offer information about applying these interventions in a wide variety of health care settings. Separate chapters on specific risk factors such as exercise, smoking, diet, and stress provide methods to help patients adopt and maintain lifestyle changes. The application of cardiovascular risk reduction strategies provided in these chapters is drawn largely from the experience gained in a research project funded by the National Heart, Lung, and Blood Institute of the National Institutes of Health. The program, known as MULTIFIT (multiple risk factor intervention), is designed to facilitate patients' recovery in the first year following a myocardial infarction.

We developed this monograph to present skills for health care professionals working with cardiovascular patients in a number of health care settings such as hospitals and cardiac rehabilitation programs. The primary focus is on patients with established coronary heart disease, specifically those who have just experienced a myocardial infarction or who are undergoing angioplasty or coronary artery surgery. However, many of the principles covered can be applied to patients at high risk for developing cardiovascular disease.

Among the unique features of this monograph are the forms and patient-related materials that are provided to facilitate management of lifestyle changes. Lifestyle modification is a challenge; we hope that this monograph increases your success in caring for patients with cardiovascular disease.

Acknowledgments

We would like to thank our many colleagues who have helped us develop lifestyle modification programs for patients with coronary heart disease. Special thanks to Dr. William Haskell and Kathy Berra, RN, BSN, who helped us conduct early studies of exercise training and who have collaborated with us since the mid-1970s; to Patti Barbarowicz, RN, MSN, who understood the value of educating this population and, through her leadership, developed the first AHA Active Partnership Program; to Dr. Albert Bandura, the father of social cognitive learning theory, who taught us the importance of self-efficacy in understanding health behavior change and to Dr. Craig Ewart who collaborated with us on our first self-efficacy studies; to Dr. Charles Dennis and many of the other cardiology fellows who actively conducted research with us through the Stanford Cardiac Rehabilitation Program (SCRP); to Dr. Kent Burnett who helped us develop some of our first computer-assisted learning programs; to Dr. Helena Kraemer and Dr. Ghassan Ghandour for their knowledge and guidance in research design, methodology, and statistics; and to Emily Clark, RD, MPH, whose expertise in nutrition and health education has allowed us to explore new avenues for health communication through computers and multimedia projects.

We are indebted to those who collaborated with us in the development and implementation of the MULTIFIT Research Program including Drs. Charles Dennis, Randal Thomas, and Robert Superko; the research nurses whose hours of dedication to patient care ensured the success of this program; and most importantly to Lynda Fisher, our operations administrator who has worked with us since 1976 and who played a key role in the conduct of this research project. We also owe our gratitude to the physicians of the Kaiser Permanente Health Care Plan for their years of support and collaboration in conducting research through the SCRP.

We pay special tribute to Denise Myers, RN, MPH, Dr. David Sobel, and Dr. Stan Tillinghast for helping us acheive our dream of moving research into clinical practice through implementation of the MULTIFIT Program as a clinical service within Kaiser Permanente Medical Centers. We thank Dr. Paul Fardy for asking us to develop this monograph and for his review and critique. Our sincere appreciation also goes to Debi Hooke and Sam Moreau for their assistance and timely work in the preparation of this manuscript.

Most importantly, we give special thanks to Dr. Robert F. DeBusk, our colleague, mentor, and friend, whose support and far-reaching vision of cardiac rehabilitation have allowed us to explore innovative, exciting, and comprehensive approaches to lifestyle management.

Chapter 1

Introduction
to Lifestyle Management

M aintaining a healthy lifestyle is difficult for even the dedicated coronary heart disease patient. Changes are problematic in a society that enjoys food, leisure, and other habits that directly affect health. Yet with the appropriate tools and with support from health care providers, patients can make changes that improve their long-term health.

It is well known that modifying coronary risk factors following a coronary heart disease (CHD) event may have a favorable impact on both morbidity and mortality. Cessation of smoking, for example, has been shown to decrease rates of reinfarction and death within one year of quitting (Sparrow & Dawber, 1978). When subjected to meta-analysis, data from secondary prevention trials directed at lowering cholesterol using diet and drugs show a 25% reduction in nonfatal myocardial infarctions (MI) (Rossouw, Lewis, & Rifkind, 1990). Moreover, recent multifactorial risk-reduction trials in patients with established CHD show a significant effect on the rate of progression of atherosclerosis (Blankenhorn et al., 1987; Blankenhorn et al., 1993; Watts et al., 1992), with hard clinical coronary events being reduced in some studies (Haskell et al., 1994; Pitt et al., 1994). The contribution to secondary prevention of lipid-lowering has also been shown to be highly cost-effective (Choudhary et al., 1984).

While the evidence clearly shows that modifying one's lifestyle is often beneficial, most people find it difficult to discard lifelong habits and to adopt and maintain unfamiliar practices. Without effective education and counseling, appropriate skills, the support of family and friends, and continued feedback and reinforcement, the likelihood of successfully changing one's lifestyle may be small, even for patients who risk a repeated coronary event.

Yet exciting knowledge and success have been acquired in the area of lifestyle management during the past two decades. Much has been learned about managing addictive behaviors, about the problems associated with relapse, and about the elements of behavioral therapy that are critical to the maintenance of beneficial behaviors. We will discuss many of these techniques in this monograph.

During the 20-year life of the Stanford Cardiac Rehabilitation Program (SCRP), our research has evolved from focusing on the role of exercise in rehabilitation to the broader issue of overall cardiovascular risk reduction and lifestyle management in patients with coronary heart disease. The change in direction reflects changes in the field as a whole. In the 1960s and 1970s, when much less was known about the safety of exercise in patients with coronary heart disease, it was necessary to determine whether patients could return to customary activity levels after many days of bed rest in a coronary care unit. Since that time, however, the field has expanded as more has been learned about all aspects of recovery and the importance each plays in ensuring a more complete recovery for the patient. The evolution of research conducted within the SCRP is a prime example of how years of experience help us to better understand the elements necessary to ensure the complete rehabilitation of patients. The remainder of this chapter presents a brief historical overview of the SCRP and its work on risk reduction for CHD patients.

Exercise Testing

The SCRP was formed as a research unit to study the natural history of patients who had experienced a myocardial infarction. A group of multidisciplinary investigators under the direction of Dr. Robert F. DeBusk and Dr. William L. Haskell conducted early research to determine the value and safety of early exercise testing in low-risk patients suffering a myocardial infarction. At that time it was almost unheard of to conduct exercise testing in a population of CHD patients only three weeks after the event. We began with symptom-limited exercise tests in low-risk post-MI patients, comparing the effects of treadmill testing with ambulatory monitoring to determine the incidence of myocardial ischemia and arrhythmias (Markiewicz, Houston, & DeBusk, 1977). The demonstration that patients without complications could undergo exercise testing at 3, 5, 7, 9, and 11 weeks after the event with no negative events laid the groundwork for a second series of studies of early exercise training in this population in the late 1970s.

In an initial study we tested the safety and efficacy of post-MI patients exercising at home beginning at 3 weeks. Patients were asked to exercise for a period of 30 minutes, 5 days per week (DeBusk, Houston, Haskell, Parker, & Fry, 1979). We knew that this population needed some form of contact with a health care professional to ensure both safety and adherence, and the telephone emerged as an important tool for follow-up. Home-based telephone follow-up and intervention has since become a vital aspect of most of our interventions. A randomized and controlled trial compared the efficacy of unsupervised home exercise training to supervised gymnasium training in the post-MI population. Home training was as effective as supervised training in increasing the functional capacity of this low-risk population, and no untoward events occurred (Miller, Haskell, Berra, & DeBusk, 1984).

Psychological Aspects of Recovery

In the late 1970s and early 1980s we also began to study the psychological aspects of recovery. These companion studies investigated the natural history of depression, anxiety, and self-efficacy in this population. We found that most patients recover relatively quickly without significant psychological problems.

Continued depression and anxiety do relate to overall recovery and problems with adherence, however.

Al Bandura, the father of social cognitive theory, became an important collaborator in our research. Our early studies of self-efficacy (Ewart, Taylor, Reese, & DeBusk, 1983; Taylor, Bandura, Ewart, Miller, & DeBusk, 1985) had demonstrated the importance of measuring the patient's confidence. For example, we found that self-efficacy levels were a better predictor of patients' physical ability than was the actual capacity achieved on treadmill exercise testing (Ewart et al., 1983). A chapter in this monograph has been devoted to these important psychological aspects of recovery.

Smoking Cessation

In the mid-1980s we began to apply our knowledge in programs to help post-MI patients quit smoking. Social cognitive theory again strongly influenced the nature of our lifestyle interventions and self-efficacy assessment formed the basis for a relapse prevention program. This antismoking intervention was behaviorally oriented and managed by nurses, and was conducted at the bedside soon after MI (Taylor, Miller, Killen, & DeBusk, 1990).

Diet Management

Based on our success in the areas of exercise and smoking, we began to test the value of managing diet in the general population. We were given the opportunity to study the efficacy of a worksite health promotion program for the PepsiCo Foundation; this allowed us to begin developing a unique dietary system. Knowing that little time was available for intervention at the worksite, we began to take advantage of computer technology. We developed a system to assess the fat and cholesterol content of individual food items and then used this data to create a computer-generated nutrition progress report. The report identified the individual food items that contributed the most fat and cholesterol to a person's diet and suggested changes. The assessment and feedback program was accompanied by a videotape and workbook. Since that time, the system has been expanded and tested in numerous patient populations. It has resulted in dietary changes producing a 7% reduction in total cholesterol (Miller, Wagner, & Rogers, 1988), an amount equal to that achieved in many of the dietary trials conducted to lower cholesterol (Hunninghake et al., 1993). Computer technology enabled us to conduct successful applications without intensive contact between health care professionals and patients.

Patient Education

Early in our research we recognized the need to provide cost-effective patient education. In 1978, members of the SCRP worked with Pat Barbarowicz, RN,

MSN, to develop and evaluate the initial American Heart Association slide/tape series "An Active Partnership for the Health of Your Heart" (Barbarowicz, Nelson, DeBusk, & Haskell, 1980). Our early home-based exercise training studies incorporated a slide/tape show; in later studies we developed videotapes, audiotapes, and workbooks to educate patients. Also at this time, Mia Clark, RD, MPH, a program nutritionist, developed DietCoach™, an interactive laser disk program for nutrition information and behavior modification.

In addition to studying rehabilitation, we have examined many other methods and issues affecting lifestyle change. We have learned much from our close involvement with the community activities of the Stanford Five-Cities Project, a long-term study examining the effects of community-wide health education on the reduction of cardiovascular disease (Farquhar et al., 1990). We have examined methods of smoking cessation (Gottlieb, Killen, Marlatt, & Taylor, 1987; Killen, Maccoby, & Taylor, 1984; Sallis, Hill, et al., 1986), weight loss and nutrition improvement (Burnett, Magel, Harrington, & Taylor, 1989; Burnett, Taylor, & Agras, 1985; Burnett, Taylor, & Agras, 1992; Fortmann, Taylor, Flora, & Winkleby, 1993; Graham, Taylor, Hovell, & Siegel, 1983; Taylor, Fortmann, et al., 1991), exercise adherence (Gossard et al., 1986; Juneau et al., 1987; King, Haskell, Taylor, Kraemer, & DeBusk, 1991; King, Taylor, Haskell, & DeBusk, 1988; Mueller et al., 1986), and stress management (Agras, Taylor, Kraemer, Southam, & Schneider, 1987). Such studies have given us experience in a broad range of lifestyle management techniques.

These 20 years of clinical research into the value of single interventions culminated in a randomized clinical study of multiple risk factors in post-MI patients, a program known as MULTIFIT (DeBusk et al., 1994). This 3-year study was funded by the National Heart, Lung, and Blood Institute of the NIH and was conducted at the Kaiser Permanente Medical Centers in the San Francisco Bay Area; it was completed in 1991. MULTIFIT incorporates a nurse case management approach to cardiovascular risk reduction, focusing on exercise training, smoking cessation, and dietary and drug management of hyperlipidemia. Nurses begin to work with patients 2 to 3 days after they are admitted to the hospital following a CHD event, and continue to work with them for one year. The majority of education and counseling is conducted by telephone rather than in face-to-face visits.

The success of the MULTIFIT program in the five hospitals studied led to its wider dissemination. It now functions as a service program in numerous Kaiser Permanente Medical Centers in northern California. Many of the tools described in the following chapters have been successfully applied in MULTIFIT and in the other studies mentioned previously. We hope they can be used to help CHD patients in other settings as well.

Stress Management

More controversial, but equally important in lifestyle management, is the adoption of a successful approach for coping with stress. Thus, in addition to the MULTIFIT program, this monograph presents a model for stress management.

During the past two decades we have been able to observe the impact of lifestyle changes on coronary heart disease. Exercising regularly, quitting smoking, maintaining a low-fat diet, and adhering to lipid-lowering medications if needed, favorably affect long-term morbidity and mortality in CHD patients (Pitt et al., 1994; Sparrow & Dawber, 1978; Watts et al., 1992). We hope that all health care professionals will meet the challenge of educating and counseling patients, providing them the skills to improve their health and well-being.

Chapter 2

Lifestyle Management: Theories of Intervention

How can health care professionals help people initiate and maintain lifestyle change? In the past 20 years much has been learned about how to institute and develop behavioral programs that can help patients with coronary heart disease adopt a healthy lifestyle.

The lifestyle change programs developed at the Stanford Cardiac Rehabilitation Program have drawn most heavily from social cognitive theory and behavior therapy and have combined theory with practical application. This chapter reviews these theories and describes how we have incorporated them into our practice.

Social Cognitive Theory

Social cognitive theory, as developed by Bandura (1977), is one of the most influential models of human behavior change. The interventions of the Multifactorial Risk Factor Intervention Trial (MRFIT) (Multiple Risk Factor Intervention Trial, 1982), the Stanford Five-Cities Project (Farquhar et al., 1990), and the Coronary Primary Prevention Trial (CPPT) (The Lipid Research Clinic, 1984), all of which encouraged people to make sustained behavior changes, were designed, in part, using social cognitive theory. In social cognitive theory, three factors are seen as influencing one another: behavior, cognition and other personal factors, and the environment. The relative influence of these three factors varies from one activity to another and from one person to another, but each factor must be considered in developing a behavior change program. For example, exercise behavior is influenced by a number of personal factors (expected and realized benefit, physiological effects, medical limitations, previous history of exercise) and by the environment (weather, facilities, social support). The relative influence of each factor may even vary from one day to the next. The optimal lifestyle change program takes all three factors into account and ensures that each contributes positively to the desired outcome.

Social cognitive theory also focuses on how people learn. Although lifestyle change is a process of behavior change, the change represents a process of learning. This is a complex process: old habits may need to be discarded and new ones adopted; the patient must learn not only how, but why, to change; people learn in different ways and at different speeds; and people are more ready to learn at one time than another. To alter their lifestyles, people may need to give up behaviors that have been firmly established. An average smoker who has smoked a pack a day for 20 years, for example, may have taken 1.5 million puffs, many of them associated with very pleasant and comforting events and feelings. Diet changes are also difficult to make. Our eating habits are strongly influenced by our parents and families, by the availability of foods, by the commercial promotion of high-fat fast foods, and by our own biological and psychological responses to eating.

Yet people can change in dramatic and sustained ways. Sometimes a heart attack, coronary bypass surgery, or angioplasty is enough to inspire dramatic lifestyle changes: a sedentary smoker with a high-fat diet becomes a jogger, adopts a diet of less than 20% fat calories, and stops smoking. But for most, the changes are modest and short-lived. Those who make only modest changes when greater change is needed are the target group for lifestyle change programs.

Social cognitive theory emphasizes the importance of self-efficacy as a mediator of behavior change. Self-efficacy is defined as ''people's judgments of their capabilities to organize and execute courses of action required to attain designated types of performances'' (Bandura, 1986, p. 391). Thus self-efficacy, which can be likened to self-confidence, reflects a person's judgment about how successfully he or she will perform tasks. It is influenced by four principle sources of information: successful performances; vicarious experiences of others' performances; verbal persuasion and other types of social influences; and the person's perception of his or her own physiological state.

Successful performances (past and present) give us a sense of accomplishment that can affect the likelihood of adopting a new behavior. People generalize from previous failures to present acts: having failed to quit smoking once, they are discouraged from trying again; recalling their unpleasant experience of physical activity in school, they are less able to engage in a physical activity program in the present. Both failures and successes relevant to a desired behavior change must therefore be reviewed when initiating a program. Misconceptions must be corrected, new skills must be taught, and confidence must be regained or bolstered to ensure success with the new behavior.

People also learn by observing others and by following the behavior of role models. This, of course, is why athletes can receive millions of dollars for promoting products; it also means that people may benefit from participation in group-based programs, where others serve as role models for positive behavior. The Active Partnership™ program is an educational videotape and workbook series developed for the American Heart Association for patients recovering from a myocardial infarction, percutaneous coronary angioplasty, or coronary artery surgery. In it, we used a wide variety of actors and patients to illustrate behavior change, ensuring that most people hospitalized for heart disease would have a model in the program with whom they could identify. Health care professionals speaking on camera lend medical authority to the program's message.

The perceived effects of a behavior change influence the likelihood that it will be maintained. Change programs are more likely to be sustained if some benefit is perceived and dropped if the changes produce discomfort. For many lifestyle changes, there are both positive and negative effects. Participation in exercise usually produces enough positive effects to help sustain people during times when they might otherwise give up. Smoking cessation is associated with positive effects in the long term but negative ones in the short term. Of the various lifestyle changes we request people to make, dietary change is least associated with immediate, demonstrable, beneficial effects other than possible weight loss. Changes in cholesterol levels, on the other hand, can serve as strong positive reinforcement. Change and the effects of change are dynamic. It is very important, therefore, for a behavior change program to have a method for monitoring the perceived and actual biopsychosocial consequences of the patient's lifestyle change and to help the individual appreciate accomplishments and overcome discomfort, frustration, or sense of failure.

Measuring self-efficacy can provide practical information for assessing the effectiveness of programs or particular interventions. Bandura and others have found that people can make very accurate predictions of their behavior and that the more specific the behavior is, the more accurate the prediction. Thus global questions such as ''Can you exercise?'' are far less useful and predictive than, ''How confident are you that you can walk four blocks?'' For the latter type of question, the level of confidence is strongly related to the behavior; that is, people who are very confident that they can walk that far are likely to be able to do so. The level of self-efficacy can also be used to determine if a therapy is effective for an individual. For instance, a post-MI patient able to walk the equivalent of four blocks safely on a treadmill but who reports low levels of efficacy will need additional help to walk four actual blocks. We must determine, for example, if the patient is anxious, fearful, or has previously experienced chest discomfort while walking.

We have been interested in using self-efficacy for both process and outcome measurements of cardiac rehabilitation interventions. In an early study we constructed self-efficacy measures of patients' confidence with regard to walking, running, climbing, engaging in sex, lifting objects, and physical exertion. Figure 2.1 shows the changes in percentage in each of these domains after a treadmill exercise test and after counseling with a nurse and physician. The shaded boxes in Figure 2.1 represent the percentage change in confidence on each self-efficacy item after a treadmill test and before counseling. The treadmill exercise test had the greatest effect on increasing confidence with regard to activities similar to treadmill exercise (walking, stair climbing, running, and general exertion). In areas where patients could not easily extrapolate the treadmill experience to real-life situations, such as lifting objects, engaging in sex, and general physical exertion, self-efficacy was more strongly influenced by post-test counseling. The intensity and duration of patients' physical activity in the weeks following the treadmill exercise were more highly correlated with these self-efficacy measurements than with peak treadmill heart rate (Ewart et al., 1983). We were also interested in assessing the impact of treadmill exercise on the patient's spouse or partner. We found that wives who underwent treadmill exercise tests had

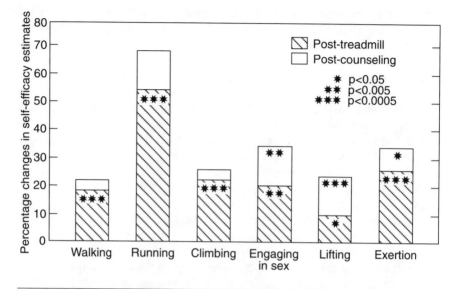

Figure 2.1   Increases in self-efficacy estimates after treadmill exercise and after counseling, compared with baseline values obtained before treadmill exercise and before counseling, respectively.

Note. From "Effects of Early Postmyocardial Infarction Exercise Testing on Self-Perception and Subsequent Physical Activity," by C.K. Ewart, C.B. Taylor, L.B. Reese, and R.F. DeBusk, 1983, *The American Journal of Cardiology*, **51**, p. 1078. Copyright 1983 by Excerpta Medica, Inc. Reprinted with permission from *The American Journal of Cardiology*.

more concordant judgements of their husbands' efficacy than spouses who did not participate.

Self-efficacy can also be used to measure outcomes. Figure 2.2 shows the results, after six months, of the global self-efficacy outcomes of 127 men participating in a group- or home-based exercise program, compared to a no-treatment control group of 37 men (DeBusk et al., 1985). The exercise group had significantly more confidence than the control group with respect to exertion, jogging, and control of tension.

Self-efficacy estimates have been developed to measure a variety of lifestyle domains. In the MULTIFIT program, we used self-efficacy estimates to conduct in-hospital assessments of patients' confidence in a number of domains following a myocardial infarction (for instance, patients' confidence to follow their medication prescription or recognize angina), to assess smoking self-efficacy in specific high-relapse situations, and to assess confidence to follow various dietary behaviors. Figure 2.3 shows the percentage of patients (N = 620) who reported greater than 70% confidence in each of six domains. The domains assessed were confidence in ability to handle stress ("Stress"); to walk a number of blocks ("Walk"); to recognize symptoms of myocardial infarction ("MI") or angina ("Angina"); to follow a low-fat, low-calorie diet ("Diet"); and to adhere to medications ("Medications").

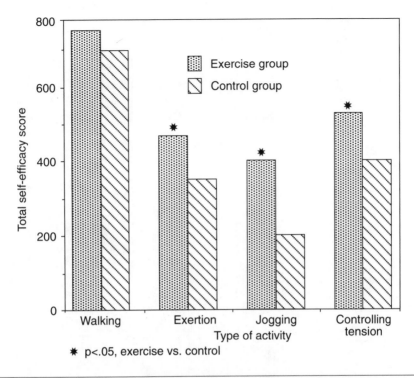

Figure 2.2 Global self-efficacy outcomes of men participating in an exercise program compared to a no-treatment control group.

We found that individuals with confidence levels greater than 70% for a particular area were unlikely to have problems in that area. For instance, a person who is more than 70% confident that he or she can adhere to a particular medication program is likely to do so. However, as is evident in Figure 2.3, about half of the subjects in the MULTIFIT program reported levels of confidence lower than 70% when they were assessed in the hospital for all lifestyle domains except confidence to follow medication prescriptions, which was very high.

Behavior Therapy

The goal of social cognitive therapy is the acquisition of knowledge and skills. Lifestyle change programs seek to promote the application of such knowledge and skills in concrete behavior changes. For many years, behavior therapists have been refining the procedures most useful for sustaining behavior change (Goldfried & Davison, 1976; Watson & Tharp, 1981). Some of these principles derive from social learning theory. However, as the name implies, behavior therapy focuses on behavior and the factors that sustain it. In recent years, cognitive factors have also become an important aspect of behavior therapy. The

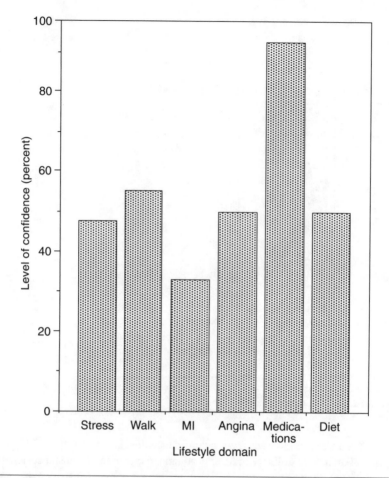

Figure 2.3 Percentage of patients who reported greater than 70% confidence in 6 domains: stress ("Stress"), confidence to walk a number of blocks ("Walk"), confidence to recognize symptoms of angina ("Angina") or myocardial infarction ("MI"), confidence to adhere to medications ("Medications"), and confidence to follow a low-fat, low-calorie diet ("Diet").

elements of successful behavior change described below are derived mainly from behavior therapy.

Relapse Prevention

The relapse prevention model focuses on preventing patients' return to old habits. It was developed by psychologist Alan Marlatt (Marlatt & Gordon, 1985) based on his work with alcoholic patients. He noted that the probability of relapse increases when an individual fails to cope adequately with a problem. Marlatt distinguishes between a lapse (a partial step back to the behavior the patient is trying to avoid) and a relapse (a more or less complete return to the undesired behavior). The failure to cope effectively leads to decreased self-efficacy, and eventually to actual relapse. Once a patient lapses, he or she experiences a "cognitive-affective" reaction that Marlatt called the Abstinence Violation Effect (Marlatt & Gordon, 1985). This effect is characterized by a sense of conflict and guilt associated with the lapse and a tendency to attribute the lapse to personal failure. This combination of guilt and self-blame increases the probability that the lapse will escalate into a full-blown relapse (see Figure 2.4). The model has particular usefulness in dealing with addictions where the urges to lapse are often pronounced and strongly connected with the lapse. The MULTIFIT smoking cessation intervention, described in more detail in chapter 8, was strongly influenced by the relapse prevention model.

Other Theories

Other lifestyle change theories have also contributed to the effectiveness of our intervention programs. Marshall Becker has long emphasized the importance of beliefs in behavior change (Becker, 1974). In the Health Belief Model, he notes that individuals are likely to change when they believe they are at risk to develop a problem, when they believe the recommended changes will improve their

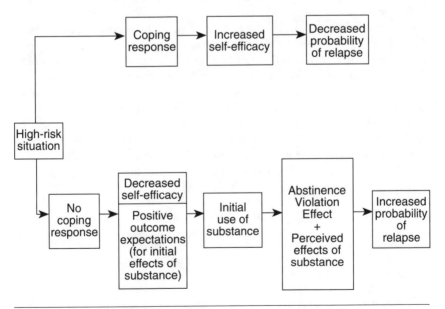

Figure 2.4 Cognitive-behavioral model of the relapse process.
Note. From "Relapse Prevention: A Self-Control Program for the Treatment of Addictive Behaviors," by G.A. Marlatt. In *Adherence, Compliance and Generalization in Behavioral Medicine* (p. 338) by R.B. Stuart (Ed.), 1982, New York: Brunner/Mazel. Reprinted with permission from Brunner/Mazel, Inc.

condition or reduce their risk, and when they believe they have the ability and resources to accomplish the desired changes. When developing a lifestyle change program, it is important to discuss the following issues with each patient for each behavior to be changed:

1. Why the patient is at risk
2. How the recommended changes will improve the patient's condition or reduce the patient's risk
3. Whether the patient has the confidence and resources to accomplish the change

Prochaska and DiClemente (1983) have noted different stages of readiness to change. Based on their observations of smokers, they have defined these stages as precontemplation, contemplation, and action. In the precontemplation stage, the individual is considering changing, but is not strongly committed to do so. In the contemplation stage, the person is willing to change and can be influenced to do so. In the action stage, the person is highly committed to changing and has begun to change. It is very helpful to know a person's level of commitment to change. If a person is uninterested in changing, the lifestyle program should be directed at changing his or her mind (or on accepting the fact that he or she does not want to change). On the other hand, the health care professional may not need to spend a great deal of time with a person already highly committed to change.

Readiness to change can be assessed fairly easily by simply asking a patient if he or she intends to undertake a particular action. A patient can be asked to use a scale of 0 to 8 (where 0 = no intention and 8 = absolute intention) to rate his or her intention to adopt a particular behavior. We find, for instance, that people with little or no intention to quit smoking are unlikely to do so, and we focus our effort on the people who have some intention of quitting. However, people's intentions are constantly changing. A person very reluctant to stop smoking one day may be willing to do so the next; a person who deplores exercise may be seen jogging next month! Therefore, do not hesitate to ask those people unwilling to change at one point about their interest in doing so, even 1 week later.

Elements of a Successful Behavioral Program

These theories and our experience in the Stanford Cardiac Rehabilitation Program have led to the following principles of rehabilitation program design (based on Taylor & Miller, 1992; Taylor & Miller, 1993; and Miller & Taylor, 1995).

1. Build positive and accurate expectations about results. A person may know how to do something (high self-efficacy and skills) but be unlikely to follow it because of low expectancy of positive results. The probability that a patient will successfully change his or her behavior and maintain that change is influenced by the accuracy and concreteness of his or her expectations. For instance, patients may adopt a low-fat diet because they think that doing so will have long-term benefits. Yet if they expect the diet to reduce their blood cholesterol level by 20%, and a reduction of only 5% is achieved, they are likely to become discouraged and may not continue to comply with the diet. The inaccuracy of their expectations led to disappointment and eventual noncompliance.

Expectations must also be concrete and understandable. Physicians and health care professionals understand the importance of weighing risk factors, but the notion of a risk factor is too abstract for many patients to understand unless the information is provided in terms that are readily applicable to their situation. For instance, it is easy for MI patients to understand that smoking doubles their chance of experiencing another heart attack; the notion that smoking increases their absolute risk by 5 to 10% may be less meaningful. Patients also respond better to immediate benefits than to long-term ones. For instance, adoption of a low-fat diet has the immediate benefit of weight loss. This is often more appealing to a patient than is the reduction of his or her risk of a heart attack by a few percentage points. Like self-efficacy, expectations are influenced by the information and instruction provided by an authority, by models, and by previous experience. Health care professionals can assess patients' expectations by asking questions such as: "What do you think will happen if you eat less meat?" Patients' answers to such questions can reveal unanticipated areas of misinformation.

2. Precisely define the behavior to be changed. Global recommendations such as "adopt a low-fat diet," "lose weight," or "exercise more" are rarely useful unless they are accompanied by specific instructions on how to change the behavior. Specific information can be presented through videotapes or pamphlets (see chapter 3). In many behavior change programs, self-observation instruments are used to help define the behaviors that need to be changed.

3. Help patients set realistic goals. Achieving a goal reinforces the maintenance of positive behavior while failure leads to discouragement and possible relapse, so it is important for health care professionals to help patients set achievable goals. Patients should be encouraged to establish goals that are realistic in terms of the magnitude and rapidity of expected change. For instance, because patients should not lose more than 0.5 to 1 kg (1 to 2 lbs) of weight per week, a patient who needs to lose 13.5 kg (30 lbs) may require 15 to 30 weeks to meet the goal. To achieve such long-term objectives, it is often helpful to have patients set intermediate goals. For example, a patient could be encouraged to lose 4.5 kg (10 lbs) over an 8-week period instead of 13.5 kg (30 lbs) over a 25- to 30-week period. The patient's likelihood of reaching a goal can be assessed using self-efficacy questions such as, "On a scale of 0 to 100 (0 = no confidence and 100 = absolute confidence), how likely are you to be able to lose 10 lbs in 3 months?" If patients are less than 70% confident that they can achieve the goal, they are unlikely to do so. The goal and/or the method of achieving it must then be modified to enhance success and confidence.

4. Use contracts to enhance commitment. Written contracts between the patient and a family member, a friend, or a health care professional can help the patient maintain behavior changes and continue with a program. Written agreements can also help enhance or clarify commitment. The agreement outlines what can be expected of the patient and what the patient can expect from the staff in return. The contract should be realistic and achievable, and should be written cooperatively with the patient. Other incentives, such as rewards patients give themselves for goals achieved, can also enhance commitment.

5. Prepare for lapses and relapses. Relapse prevention, as discussed earlier, is a method to help patients avoid returning to old habits. The principles of relapse prevention are: (a) to identify situations, feelings, or events where lapse or relapse may occur; (b) to develop skills to cope with these situations; (c) to practice these skills; and (d) to continue to monitor threats to lapse or relapse, developing and implementing strategies to deal with these new situations as needed.

6. Model the desired behavior. Patients often understand better and are more motivated to change if they can observe a desired behavior being modeled by others. A variety of videotapes is available for modeling behaviors such as preparing low-fat foods, requesting special menus in restaurants, and asking a family member or friend not to smoke in one's home.

7. Use prompts to remind the patient of the desired behavior. If a new behavior requires practice, prompting it can be helpful. Prompts can be as simple as a sticker on the patient's watch or telephone, a chart on the refrigerator, or a note in a datebook. Telephone prompting programs can be used to remind patients about appointments, medications, and exercising.

8. Provide feedback about the patient's progress. Feedback strongly influences behavior change. From a behavioral standpoint, feedback should focus on the behaviors undergoing change as well as on the desired final outcome. The behavioral variables include exercise adherence, confidence to cope with smoking urges, avoidance of high-fat foods, taking medications. These behaviors, rather than the results they are meant to produce, should be the primary source of feedback, although tests (such as periodic treadmill tests, serum cholesterol levels, and weight measurement) that reflect the success of these behavioral changes are also important sources of feedback.

9. Teach problem solving. Most behavior therapists use a problem-solving approach to help patients overcome difficulties in changing their health behavior. The problem-solving approach is comprised of six basic steps:

1. Specify the problem to be solved in concrete, specific terms.
2. Identify possible solutions.
3. Develop a plan for implementing these solutions.
4. Test the solutions.
5. Evaluate the results.
6. Repeat the process if the initial solutions have not been successful.

10. Reward achievement. Positive reinforcement has a very strong influence on behavior. For this reason, many behavioral programs include monetary, interpersonal, or accomplishment rewards. Patients are rarely successful in developing and implementing a reward system on their own. A reward system requires help and monitoring from a health care professional or someone else in the patient's social network.

Feedback that increases the likelihood that a behavior will continue is one important source of positive reinforcement. Many kinds of feedback can provide reinforcement, including verbal feedback (e.g., praise from a health care professional), physiological feedback (e.g., being able to run farther as one becomes more fit), a sense of accomplishment (e.g., for having achieved a goal), monetary or symbolic rewards (e.g., a T-shirt for participating in an exercise class), and cognitive feedback (what patients tell themselves about their progress). Of course, for feedback and reinforcement to occur, the patient's behavior must be monitored. The use of simple monitoring tools and telephone calls can provide opportunities for feedback and reinforcement.

11. Enlist appropriate social support as needed. Social isolation has been associated with increased mortality from coronary heart disease (Ruberman, Weinblatt, Goldberg, & Chaudhary, 1984). Spousal involvement in an exercise program may result in greater concordance of expectations and may therefore reduce conflict between patient and spouse (Taylor et al., 1985). A buddy system (e.g., nonsmokers helping smokers with cessation) may improve the patient's compliance with the lifestyle change program. Encouraging active participation by spouses, friends, and family members is an important element of a successful behavior change program.

These 11 principles have guided all of our lifestyle interventions and have been incorporated into the management of diet in the MULTIFIT program for post-MI patients (see the "Hyperlipidemic Diet Intervention for MULTIFIT," p. 19). When designing a lifestyle change program, it is important to keep in mind the socioeconomic and ethnic characteristics of the target group. Materials should be appropriate to the culture, education, and values of that group. In many programs, far too much of the available effort is put into the front end of behavior change programs, and far too little into the ongoing issues related to sustaining behavior change.

Responsibility

Our model is directive, and might be accused of not giving patients enough responsibility for changes in their own lifestyle. Some argue that patients must take responsibility for such changes and must learn to sustain them by making their own choices. Certainly self-initiated change is more likely to be sustained than change encouraged by an outside force. Yet is the individual really able to freely choose healthy habits in today's society? Many powerful forces make such a choice difficult: smokers are more than likely to be addicted to tobacco, an addiction encouraged by billions of advertising dollars; those who do not smoke may still be forced to work in smoke-filled environments; fatty fast foods are cheap, tasty, and ubiquitous; many communities lack public spaces conducive to exercise. Thus while the self-initiative and determination of the patient should be supported wherever possible, the direction, knowledge, and authority of the health care professional are important forces for lifestyle change.

Of course, the patient holds ultimate responsibility for making changes in his or her lifestyle. This message must be made clear in lifestyle change programs, though the patient should not be blamed for failure to change. Health care professionals provide the tools, the support, the positive reinforcement, the opportunity for change, and the ongoing support the patient needs to sustain the changes he or she has made. In the last analysis, health care professionals are partners in the lifestyle change process.

Summary

Social cognitive theory and self-efficacy analysis are the most widely recognized approaches to health behavior change. Other models and theories, such as the relapse prevention model and the health belief model, provide important additional insights and can be used to make intervention programs more effective. By incorporating the basic principles discussed in this chapter, health care professionals can help patients adopt and maintain significant lifestyle changes.

Hyperlipidemic Diet Intervention for MULTIFIT

Build positive and accurate expectations about results.

- Nurses meet with post-MI patients in hospital to discuss the importance of dietary change.
- A workbook reviews reasons/benefits for lowering serum cholesterol.
- The AHA Active Partnership™ diet video provides an overview of the benefits of dietary change.

Precisely define the behavior to be changed.

- Assess baseline fat and cholesterol intake using a semiquantitative food frequency questionnaire (FFQ).
- Assess self-efficacy to make dietary changes.

Help patients set realistic goals.

- Three weeks after the infarction, the patient and his or her spouse or partner meet with a program nurse to set goals using feedback from an individualized progress summary sheet generated by computer from their FFQ.

Use contracts to enhance commitment.

- Patient signs a written agreement to participate in the MULTIFIT program. The patient's efficacy to continue dietary changes is assessed during each maintenance encounter.

Prepare for lapses and relapses.

- Counseling session at 3 months focuses on identifying possible situations where the patient may lapse from the diet.
- At 6 months, the patient is given a self-monitoring form to monitor progress toward his or her dietary goals. The form includes tips for handling situations that present a high risk for lapse.

Model the desired behavior.

- The Active Partnership™ videotape provides role models for desired behaviors.

Use prompts to remind the patient of the desired behavior.

- Telephone calls occur at monthly intervals during the first 3 months to determine patient's success in meeting goals, to address lapses, and to answer questions relative to diet.

Provide feedback about the patient's progress.

- Patients complete two additional FFQs and are given a computer-generated progress summary report providing feedback about dietary changes and success in reaching goals. The progress summary report is discussed in follow-up telephone calls.
- Serum cholesterol is measured at 60, 90, 180, and 360 days.

Teach problem solving.

- Problem-solving techniques are taught in each face-to-face meeting and each telephone contact. Telephone algorithms include problem-solving guidelines.

Reward achievement.

- Positive changes in diet are reinforced by the nurses, by the computerized reports, and by reductions in serum lipids.

Enlist appropriate social support as needed.

- Nurses and dietitians encourage the patient's significant others to attend sessions and to join in telephone calls.
- The nurse and dietitian act as strong agents of social support for the patients.

Note. From *Rehabilitation of the Coronary Patient* (3rd ed., p. 465), by N.K. Wenger and H.K. Hellerstein (Eds.), 1992, New York: Churchill Livingstone. Reprinted with permission of Churchill Livingstone, Inc.

Chapter 3

Education, Communication, and Methods of Intervention

I n the previous chapter we reviewed the theories and principles of intervention. In this chapter we discuss issues related to implementing programs: education of patients, principles of communication, and methods of intervention.

Patient Education

Behavior change and learning are intimately connected. Health care providers must also be educators, so it is important to review some of the basic principles of teaching before planning an intervention.

Pat Comoss (1992) has designed practical guidelines for teaching cardiac rehabilitation patients. The basic principles are as follows:

1. Carefully define the learning objectives.
2. Choose the best methods to reach the objectives.
3. Prepare lessons in advance.
4. Practice delivery of lessons.
5. Emphasize self-directed learning and the patient's active involvement in the learning process.
6. Scrutinize each teaching aid for appropriateness, comprehensibility, and style. Is the information current, correct, and compatible with objectives? Is the visual style acceptable?
7. Evaluate the patient's knowledge of the subject matter. If the patient is already familiar with the subject being taught, consider more advanced materials or simply congratulate the patient on his or her knowledge of the material.
8. Consider the patient's learning style, taking into account their past experience and current practice. A person who never reads, for example, will be unlikely to read handouts or pamphlets, while a serious reader may prefer more detailed text materials.
9. Set priorities for learning objectives; differentiate between what must be learned and what should be learned.
10. Evaluate the outcome.

Learning is best accomplished when the patient is ready to learn. Being ready to learn depends on both ability and willingness. Cardiac rehabilitation professionals may make mistakes both in trying to teach something to a patient who is not ready to learn and not teaching when the patient is ready. A patient's readiness to learn can change rapidly in the course of recovery from MI or bypass surgery. Many believe that there is a "window of opportunity"—a brief, optimal time for teaching patients, usually just before discharge from the hospital, after the patient has begun to recover from the acute event, procedure, or surgery. While there are advantages to educating patients while they are still in the hospital, we believe that patients are often interested and willing to learn during the course of postdischarge recovery. However, it is also important to remember that the patient's medical status affects learning. Many patients are confused following surgery and are not able to retain information. Others are too sick to be interested in learning. By the time such patients are able to concentrate on learning, they are usually about to be discharged. In-hospital education programs must also be designed to accommodate increasingly brief in-hospital stays. Consequently, clear priorities need to be established when selecting information to be presented before discharge.

Deciding on the Content of Educational Materials

When designing a lifestyle change program, begin by selecting the topics to be covered. Be aware that prepackaged educational programs often cover information that is already familiar to some patients. To personalize instruction, Comoss (1992) asks patients to indicate the topics for which they would like more information, and to rate the importance of each topic using a 5-point scale (where 1 = least important and 5 = most important). Her list of topics includes: heart structure and function, what to do about chest pain, preparing for heart attack emergencies, the healing process, and questions about returning to work. Information is then provided only on topics of interest to the patient.

It is important to assess educational efforts periodically. This can be done by testing patients on the key ideas of their lifestyle program. The interactive learning systems discussed below provide both testing and corrective feedback in an efficient, nonthreatening manner.

Interpersonal Communication

Good communication between the patient and health care professional is essential to the effectiveness of a lifestyle program (Taylor & Houston Miller, 1993). Good communication skills are helpful both for obtaining information from an individual and for establishing a positive relationship with him or her. It is beyond the scope of this monograph to discuss the principles of good communication in depth; we can only present some basic guidelines. First, to develop a good relationship with the patient, it is important to convey a sense of empathy. Show that you care about the patient and understand what he or she is experiencing.

Health care professionals often first meet the patient when he or she is in physical pain, is afraid, dysphoric, and perhaps confused. The health care professional's sensitivity to these issues will create rapport with the patient.

Do not be judgmental. Listen carefully to the patient's beliefs, fears, and statements about symptoms. Encourage the patient to speak openly. Facilitate interactive communication by using noncommittal acknowledgments such as nodding the head, adopting an attentive posture, and commenting, "Oh, I see." Invite the patient to expand on thoughts and feelings, using statements such as, "Could I hear more?" "Please go on," or "I don't quite understand," and by paraphrasing the patient's comments. Avoid disruptive communication behaviors such as displaying anger, interrupting the patient unnecessarily, and telling him or her how to feel. Conduct yearly peer reviews using audiotapes of sessions with patients.

As a relationship develops and the health care professional learns more about the patient, it is sometimes necessary to use confrontation. Confrontation involves directing the patient's attention to something he or she may not be aware of or is reluctant to admit. When using confrontation, address only the observable facts; do not make inferences about the patient's motives or emotional state. Many health care professionals avoid confrontation and in so doing, limit their effectiveness with patients. Confrontation is sometimes avoided for fear of making patients angry. In our experience, confrontation rarely provokes anger; when it does, if the confrontation has been carried out in an appropriate manner, the anger usually indicates that the confrontation was accurate and important.

Methods of Intervention

Lifestyle change programs have relied, traditionally, on personal instruction with supplementation from print and, occasionally, videotapes. In the following section, we discuss various educational methods for behavior change.

Printed Materials

MULTIFIT uses a variety of printed materials, central to which is the Active Partnership™ workbook. In designing and developing this workbook we followed these assumptions:

- Patients will only read material of interest to them.
- The key points should be presented first and highlighted; more detailed information should be presented later, if at all.
- Most patients read only a limited amount of printed information, even if it is interesting to them and very well designed. Some health educators believe that people read only the first 10 to 15% of even a short pamphlet.
- Interested patients who want more information should be provided lengthier print pieces such as manuals, books, or pamphlets.

- Very detailed information is best presented in the many available lifestyle change books, not pamphlets.
- Present information of interest to a general audience rather than very detailed information appropriate only for a more select audience.

Each piece of material given to a patient should be checked for readability. Is the visual style acceptable? Is the print large and legible? Is the reading level in average range? That is, could the average junior high school student (grades 5 to 9) understand all the words, and if not, are more difficult words defined in simple terms? On the other hand, make sure the material is not so simple as to be offensive or meaningless. For a detailed guide to the principles of writing and print design, see the book *Everyone's Guide to Successful Publications* by Elizabeth Adler (1993).

Video

Many rehabilitation programs use videotapes to educate patients. A wide variety of videotapes, some specifically designed for patients with CHD, have been developed. There are many advantages to using video as an education tool:

- Video programs can be very engaging, holding the patient's interest and attention until the message is fully conveyed.
- Videotapes can be taken home and viewed with family members.
- Video programs can be viewed repeatedly.
- Video programs can be mass produced at relatively low cost.

The major disadvantage of video programs is the cost of development, particularly when audiences have come to expect high-quality, professionally produced, and entertaining programs. However, good video programs are available on many lifestyle change topics, and some programs have been developed specifically for patients with cardiovascular disease. We have produced a number of videotapes over the years, culminating in the Active Partnership™ videotape series. However, other excellent videotape materials are also available. Rehabilitation specialists should investigate existing videotapes before developing their own.

There has been very little evaluation of the use of videotapes for lifestyle change. One would expect videotapes to be most useful in the adoption phase of behavior change and less so in the maintenance phase. Exercise programs are a possible exception, as patients often use videotapes for regular instruction. In a controlled study, we evaluated the use of a video program developed by the Nestlé Corporation to help overweight individuals lose weight through changes in diet and exercise. Because we suspected that even patients who were highly motivated to lose weight would have difficulty adhering to the program, we supplemented the video with a second intervention that focused on helping the individuals adhere to the videotape series. Six months after completion of the program, the group receiving the video program and the supplementary intervention had lost 3.2 kg, while those receiving the video program alone had lost only 1.8 kg (Taylor & Stunkard, 1993). This suggests that the effectiveness of videotapes can be enhanced through interventions designed to improve their use.

Computers

In many areas of education, interactive, multimedia computers are beginning to replace printed materials and videos. Interactive computers contain all of the advantages of print and video while allowing for personalization. In interactive programs, the patient can control aspects of his or her interaction with the computer. Using interactive computer programs, information can be presented and tested immediately. There is a substantial body of literature demonstrating the effectiveness of computer-based instruction.

The cost of computer hardware and software has limited, until recently, the widespread use of computer-based instruction. The increasing availability of relatively inexpensive CD-ROM drives for home computers now makes it feasible for many more people to use this technology for lifestyle change.

At the present time, the most common use of computers for lifestyle change seems to be for health risk appraisal. The user answers a number of questions about such health behaviors as smoking, seat belt use, family history, and diet. The program then provides a risk assessment and recommendations for change. A single health risk appraisal may motivate individuals to make some behavior change, but without a follow-up from a health care professional it is unlikely to have a lasting impact.

Computers can be combined with print materials to integrate assessment, intervention, and management. Over the years, we have experimented with a number of formats combining print and computers. In a project funded by The PepsiCo Foundation (Miller et al., 1988) we developed a computer-generated feedback system. We sought to provide very simple but useful feedback on the patient's progress in exercise, smoking status, and diet, over the course of a year. A summary sheet was accompanied by a personalized, computer-generated letter. This system became the foundation for the Computer-Assisted Learning System (CALS) developed by the SCRP (see chapter 6). The program has also been adapted for Macintosh computers to help young people make behavior changes (Burnett et al., 1989).

In the MULTIFIT program, computers help organize and manage the intervention using algorithms that provide intervention guidelines. The computer also provides data management, scheduling, and prompting. These functions can be combined with voice mail and education. Educational materials can even be downloaded via modem to the patient's home computer.

Telephone Calls

The telephone is an effective but often underutilized tool for health care intervention. Currently, only 10% of all patient-provider telephone calls are initiated by the provider. Many face-to-face interactions can be replaced by telephone calls, which are more efficient and less costly. Because of its usefulness and wide availability, we discuss telephone interventions in some detail.

The telephone can help remove some of the barriers to health care encountered by the patient. Telephone calls eliminate the need to travel to a facility, the burden of transportation for some, and the time wasted waiting to see a physician. Furthermore, when surveillance of symptoms becomes critically important, especially in cases of chronic disease such as CHD, telephone follow-up allows for increased contact between patients and health care providers.

Many studies of CHD patients have demonstrated the potential of the telephone. It can be used to help patients make lifestyle changes, to enhance their psychosocial functioning, and as a method of surveillance. The use of the telephone as an intervention to increase patient knowledge and to lessen patient anxiety has been documented in randomized clinical trials in patients with CHD (Beckie, 1989; Garding, Kerr, & Bay, 1988; Pozen et al., 1977). Garding, Kerr, and Bay (1988) found that patients receiving three telephone calls by cardiac rehabilitation nurses in the eight weeks after MI had significantly more knowledge about risk factors and exercise recommendations than did those in a control group. Similarly, in a study of postcoronary artery surgery patients (Beckie, 1989), a supportive, educational telephone program carried out by nurses during the first six weeks of the patients' convalescence at home increased knowledge about coronary artery disease and related self-care measures and decreased stated anxiety levels. In this study, the patients' knowledge level was inversely correlated with their anxiety level.

The telephone has also been used successfully to improve outcomes relative to quality of life. Pozen et al. (1977) demonstrated that education, support, and follow-up telephone calls during recovery resulted in an earlier return to work and in decreased smoking in patients hospitalized within a coronary care unit, as compared to a control group. In a similar randomized trial, we utilized nurses to provide a behavioral relapse prevention intervention to smokers, incorporating telephone follow-ups in the 6 months after infarction, and achieved a biochemically confirmed cessation rate of 71% at 12 months compared to 45% in a control group (Taylor et al., 1990).

The telephone has also been used as an effective method for monitoring the safety of coronary patients initiating health behavior changes such as exercise, and as a means of surveillance of patients in the early days following a coronary heart disease event. Nicklin (1986) developed a call-back system for patients and families in which nurses responded to patients' messages within five minutes of a call. In 44% of cases, patients were advised to go to an emergency room or were directed to contact their physicians due to a change in symptomatology. The call-back system was a useful mechanism for providing feedback to the patient and his or her family, for identifying learning needs, and for reinforcing education. In a study conducted at the SCRP, we sought to establish if it was safe and effective for patients to exercise at home following a myocardial infarction. In the study, weekly telephone contact with patients during exercise training sessions resulted in a small proportion of patients being referred back to physicians for management of their symptoms; it also may have contributed to the low rate of cardiac events observed in patients who underwent home exercise training (DeBusk et al., 1985).

Practical Use of the Telephone

The telephone affords an opportunity to communicate with patients in a way similar to face-to-face visits. The telephone can be used to

- provide support and reassurance,
- answer questions,
- provide information or instruction,
- teach skills,
- collect data,
- prompt or remind patients,
- help patients solve problems in adhering to a program,
- offer feedback,
- provide positive reinforcement, and
- recommend triage or surveillance.

It is not enough simply to provide patients with a telephone number; they may hesitate to bother their physician to ask seemingly mundane questions, and are often reluctant to initiate telephone contact except in an emergency. Patients may also be reluctant to initiate telephone contact because they are embarrassed to admit they have not adhered to some aspect of their rehabilitation program. In our smoking cessation studies, for example, fewer than 10% of patients call when they are having trouble resisting the urge to smoke. For these reasons, we advise health care professionals to initiate the telephone calls.

Before one considers developing a telephone system for managing patients, it is important to consider the following: (a) What are the goals of the telephone contact (support, information, data gathering)? (b) Is the frequency of calls appropriate for the goals being pursued? (c) Should family members be involved in telephone conversations? (d) Has adequate time been allowed for each call?

Structuring Telephone Calls

When designing the structure of telephone calls, keep in mind the following five key points:

1. Determine what is to be accomplished in a telephone conversation. Will the telephone be used to obtain data, to provide support, to deliver feedback, to monitor compliance, to provide referral, to answer questions, or all of the above?
2. Determine if family members should be involved in telephone conversations. Weigh the costs and benefits of potentially longer conversations.
3. Develop good communication and interviewing skills. Be empathetic and supportive; learn to redirect the conversation firmly but politely when

necessary; know when to make a referral; and know how to terminate telephone relationships tactfully when the program is completed.

4. Script telephone calls, if appropriate, or develop a list of key points to be covered during the conversation. Structuring calls helps to focus the conversation and prevent rambling responses from patients.

5. To develop telephone skills and to become more comfortable with the procedures, conduct practice telephone conversations and tape-record them. Listening to and analyzing one's own conversations and those of others will enhance interviewing technique and general communication skills.

Carefully determine the appropriate frequency of telephone calls and avoid burdening patients and health care professionals with unnecessary calls. It is often appropriate to schedule more frequent calls during the beginning of a patient's behavior change program. We find, for example, it is important to call patients one week after the initiation of a home exercise training program to assess difficulties in initiating exercise, the presence of unusual symptoms, and the patients' feelings about the intensity of the exercise. Because most smokers relapse immediately upon hospital discharge, we believe it is important to contact the patient approximately 48 hours after discharge. In a telephone call-back system for post-MI patients during the first three months after discharge, Nicklin (1986) found that 55% of all calls from patients occurred within the first two weeks after discharge. Thus it is clearly important to support and reassure patients early in the recovery period, when they are experiencing heightened anxiety and fear. As patients move toward the maintenance stage of behavioral changes, calls to monitor adherence, to provide reminders, and to provide postitive reinforcement to patients can usually be structured at monthly or quarterly intervals.

To increase the efficiency and uniformity of our telephone interventions, we have developed a standardized telephone interview. Each segment of the phone call is connected to an algorithm. For a sample telephone questionnaire to monitor patients who have just stopped smoking, see the ''Telephone Interview for Patients Attempting to Quit Smoking'' on p. 101. A structured call ensures coverage of the appropriate information and better management of the length of telephone conversations, and can provide a method of gathering important data about both process and outcomes. If a scripted telephone interview is not appropriate, a check-off list should be used to ensure that the goals of the call are met. Unstructured calls can lead to lengthy conversations and failure to accomplish necessary tasks.

Problems Associated With Phone Calls

Some patients can be extremely needy or lonely and can take up an inordinate amount of the health care professional's time if allowed to do so. Patients who require a significant amount of time in telephone interviews may need, instead, the support of a therapy group or the help of a professional therapist. The excessive length of telephone conversations may be due, alternatively, to the interviewer's inability to discontinue a conversation. In cardiovascular risk reduction programs, we find that telephone calls for counseling purposes take an average of 10 minutes when properly structured. This includes time for responding to the patient's questions and concerns. Wasson et al. (1992) reported that clinicians estimated 10 minutes or less were required for 83% of all phone calls recorded when telephone follow-up was used as a substitute for clinic visits. When telephone calls are used to monitor patients' use of medications, or to convey information about scheduled appointments, they often take only 2 to 5 minutes or less.

One of the most difficult problems associated with telephone calls is reaching patients. To address this problem, we schedule telephone calls as we do face-to-face visits. If this is not possible, it is helpful to keep a record of the days and times when a patient can usually be reached. It is important to obtain the patient's home and work telephone numbers, as well as the number of a friend or relative who will always know the whereabouts of the patient. This facilitates access and decreases frustration in reaching patients if the telephone follow-up program is to occur over an extended period of time. Finally, one should set criteria indicating when a structured telephone call is to be defined as a "missed call." It is not cost-effective to make numerous unsuccessful attempts to reach patients. We have chosen to use three calls as the maximum number of attempts, provided a machine is available to leave a message for the patient. If the patient has not returned our call after messages have been left three times, the telephone call is considered a missed call.

In the MULTIFIT program, telephone calls are used to replace face-to-face visits, thus reducing the need for patients to return frequently to the medical care setting. Information and counseling about all areas of cardiovascular risk intervention (smoking, diet, exercise, stress), as well as symptomatology and psychosocial problems, are covered in an average 10-minute call. Telephone calls are more frequent (every one to two weeks) during the adoption stage of behavior change, and less frequent (monthly or bimonthly) during the maintenance stage. When asked to evaluate the support they received from the MULTIFIT program for making lifestyle changes, patients rated the telephone calls with nurses as the most important component.

Group Interventions

In cardiac rehabilitation, there is a long history of using groups to help patients cope with psychosocial problems, and most present-day cardiac rehabilitation programs use group-based interventions (Adsett & Bruhn, 1968; Gruen, 1975; Ibrahim, Feldman, & Sultz, 1974; Oldenburg, Perkins, & Andrews, 1985; Rahe, Ward, & Hayes, 1979). Group programs designed to deal with psychosocial problems and/or to reduce stress or Type A behavior have proven effective in reducing morbidity and mortality (Rahe et al., 1979; Friedman et al., 1984).

Group therapy has a number of advantages over individual therapy. First, groups can be more efficient because one health care professional can help a number of people at the same time. Second, group members can benefit from the experience, wisdom, feedback, and knowledge of others in the group. Third, groups can provide psychological support not only during group sessions, but in outside contacts that can last for years. Patients do not feel as alone or discouraged when they realize that others have experienced similar thoughts, feelings, and problems.

Groups have some disadvantages as well. First, it is often difficult to organize a group. This problem can be overcome by maintaining ongoing, open groups, but such groups often develop less cohesiveness. Second, attendance at a therapy group can be expensive and inconvenient; it requires regular transportation to the group and time to participate. In one study, adherence to an exercise program was significantly lower in group-based treatment when compared to home-based treatment (King et al., 1991). And finally, special skills are required to lead a therapy group. Intense emotional experiences and complex psychological problems may not be handled well in a group setting. Overall, however, groups are an excellent method of educating and supporting patients.

We have developed home-based interventions, in part, to overcome the logistical problems of groups. Home-based interventions offer the advantage of convenience and comfort but lack the valuable element of group contact. Some of this contact can be replaced by phone calls from nurses, which can serve both to monitor and facilitate behavior change and to provide social support.

Summary

Using multiple channels of communication to educate patients may facilitate the educational process. Each medium of communication—print, video, computers, and the telephone—offers distinct advantages for lifestyle change programs. To improve their effectiveness in lifestyle change interventions, health care professionals should be aware of the advantages and disadvantages of each medium and should make note of the principles discussed above.

Chapter 4

Psychological Issues Affecting Lifestyle Change

Heart attacks and cardiovascular surgery are upsetting events and can temporarily worsen preexisting psychological conditions. On the other hand, such events may lead to psychological growth, reassessment of one's values, and a commitment to a healthier lifestyle. We believe that five domains of psychological functioning—depression, anxiety, alcohol and drug abuse, social support and marital status, and stress and anger—impact changes in lifestyle; these five factors should be considered when designing a lifestyle change program. Health care professionals should be able (a) to identify individuals with problems in any of these five areas, (b) to understand how a problem in one of these areas may affect the patients' participation in a lifestyle change program, and (c) to refer the patient to other care providers for additional help as needed (Taylor & Houston Miller, 1993). Depending on the method of assessment, the population, and the setting, approximately 25 to 30% of medical patients have experienced depression or anxiety, and/or have abused alcohol (Kessler et al., 1987; Schulberg et al., 1985; Von Korff et al., 1987; Zung, 1965). The prevalence of these disorders is likely to be even higher in patients with cardiovascular disease.

Screening

A number of short, reasonably specific, and sensitive screening tests have been developed to help primary care physicians identify these problems (Meakin, 1992; Linn & Yager, 1984). In the MULTIFIT program, we use the "Psychosocial Questionnaire" (p. 38). to screen all patients while they are still in the hospital. The questions for this instrument were modified from items on existing screening tests (King, Taylor, Haskell, & DeBusk, 1989; Taylor, 1987).

The first four questions concern depression, anger, anxiety, and stress. If a patient reports a moderate to very severe level of distress on these questions (a score ≥ 5), or if the patient wants help in one of these areas (question 5), we elicit more information to determine the extent and severity of the problem. The screening questions are not meant to be diagnostic, but to indicate potential problems.

Questions 7 to 10 are taken from the CAGE Questionnaire and are used to screen for potential alcohol abuse (Ewing, 1984). "CAGE" stands for Cut down, Annoyed, Guilt, and Eye-opener. A "yes" response to any of these questions may indicate alcohol abuse. Two or more "yes" responses indicate an increased probability of past or present alcohol abuse. The amount of alcohol consumed should also be assessed and the patient should be asked about use of any illegal drugs. The interviewer should also inquire about medical abnormalities that may reflect alcohol abuse, such as peptic ulcer, gastrointestinal disease, or elevated liver enzymes. It is important to remember that most patients abusing alcohol under-report their alcohol use. Alcohol abuse has both a consumption and a behavioral component; the latter is often more telling than the former. The health care professional suspicious of alcohol abuse should determine how much the patient is motivated to drink despite their own best interests. For instance, even an occasional drinker may have a serious drinking problem if his or her drinking results in family problems, difficulties at work, or other social problems.

Questions 13 and 14 are used to screen for inadequate social support. Many intricate and lengthy instruments have been developed to assess this complex domain. Instruments must determine the type (financial, physical, social) and extent of support needed, the difference between available support and support that is actually used, and many other factors. Our questionnaire focuses on whether or not patients live alone, a factor which has been shown to predict subsequent mortality following an MI; we also ask who helps the patient at home. The latter question is useful for identifying patients who have little or no help yet need it. In previous clinical research trials, we have assessed satisfaction with marriage, work, and other domains. While troubles in these domains are common, they often remain stable in the course of rehabilitation and have not proven to be predictive of the outcome of rehabilitation (Taylor, 1987). We have therefore removed these items from our baseline screening.

Table 4.1 reports data on 470 males and 150 females participating in the MULTIFIT program in one of four Kaiser Permanente Medical Centers (respondents who answered yes to one of the CAGE questions were considered to have

Table 4.1   Percentages of Post-MI Patients Reporting Significant Psychosocial Problems in Hospital

	Males (n = 470)	Females (n = 150)
Moderate to severe depression	10.2%	14%
Moderate to severe anxiety	13%	24%
Significant problems with anger	13%	15%
Moderate to severe stress	22%	26%
Problems with alcohol	20%	9%

possible problems with alcohol). The table shows the percentages of patients who demonstrated moderate to severe depression, anxiety, or stress; dissatisfaction with social support; and problems with alcohol or anger. It is clear that a significant number of post-MI patients experience serious psychosocial problems.

Depression

Depression affects 5 to 10% of adults at one time or another and occurs in 10 to 20% of post-MI patients (Shuster, Stern, & Tesar, 1992; Taylor, DeBusk, Davidson, Houston, & Burnett, 1981). Depression is a serious problem and may even affect morbidity and mortality (Eaker, 1989). The main symptoms of depression include emotional problems such as depressed mood, feeling blue, irritability, anxiety, loss of interest, withdrawal from others, and preoccupation with death; cognitive problems such as feeling worthless or guilty, hopelessness, despair, poor concentration, indecisiveness, and suicidal feelings; and vegetative problems such as fatigue, lack of energy, trouble sleeping, loss of appetite, weight loss or gain, lack of interest in sex, and looking depressed. The level of depression can be assessed with self-report instruments such as the Beck Depression Inventory (Beck, Ward, Mendelson, Mock, & Erbaugh, 1961) or the Zung Depression Scale (Zung, 1965), or with a structured interview such as the Hamilton Rating Scale for Depression (Hamilton, 1960). Of these, the Beck inventory is the most widely used. A score of greater than 10 is generally considered to indicate a level of depression needing further evaluation. Of course, many of these symptoms are also characteristic of patients with heart disease.

It is not surprising that a cardiac event such as a myocardial infarction can exacerbate depression. Depression is related to real or anticipated loss, and the life-threatening situation of heart disease brings about actual and perceived losses in most aspects of a person's life, at least temporarily. Whether this perceived or actual loss leads to sustained depression depends on the patient's personality, personal and social resources, coping mechanisms, and medical treatment. It also appears that some people have a biological predisposition to depression. For them, the onset of depression may be gradual and difficult to detect. Some of the medications used to treat patients with cardiovascular disease may also cause depression or symptoms that mimic depression. For instance, between 10 and 35% of patients on beta-blockers experience depression or other symptoms of psychological distress (Petruzzello, Landers, Hatfield, Kubitz, & Salazar, 1991).

Helping Patients With Depression

Several factors influence the health care provider's ability to help patients with depression. Timing is one important factor. The best time to determine if further treatment for depression is necessary is after the patient has been home for about two weeks. By that time, patients have had time to adjust to their illness and to assess their progress at home. It is also important to remember that depression can hinder patients' participation in lifestyle change programs. Depressed patients may not have the energy or enthusiasm to pursue recommended changes, and patients with addictions, such as smokers, may resist change for fear of becoming depressed.

If the patient can be convinced to participate, however, lifestyle interventions can have a positive impact on depression. Lifestyle change programs can convey a sense of hope to the patient. Exercise, in particular, has consistently been shown to be a good ancillary treatment for depression (Benight & Taylor, 1994). When a patient participates in a lifestyle change program, his or her condition is more likely to be identified, making it possible for a referral to an appropriate specialist. Depression, even severe depression, is a readily treatable condition. Modern psychopharmacologic agents combined with psychotherapy can help most patients overcome their depression in 3 to 6 months.

Anxiety

Anxiety affects everyone at one time or another (Taylor & Arnow, 1988). As shown in Table 4.1, 13% of males and 24% of females reported moderate to severe levels of anxiety while in the hospital following a myocardial infarction. Severe anxiety, however, can lead to avoidance behavior and unnecessary restrictions of life's activities; it can also be associated with severe depression and terrifying panic attacks. Acute anxiety can often be resolved with reassurance or brief periods of psychotherapy.

The measurement of anxiety is unlike the measurement of depression: quantification of anxiety with a standardized instrument is usually no more helpful than qualitative assessment based on clinical questions. However, there are a number of standardized instruments available. The most widely used is the Spielberger State-Trait Anxiety Inventory (Spielberger, 1983).

Chronic anxiety is usually a secondary condition associated with depression, but it may also represent a primary anxiety disorder. One should always test for depression when patients display anxiety. The two most prevalent primary anxiety disorders are Generalized Anxiety Disorder and Panic Disorder. Generalized Anxiety Disorder is characterized by excessive worry and signs of motor tension (e.g., trembling, muscle tension, restlessness), autonomic hyperactivity (e.g., sweating, dry mouth, and frequent urination), vigilance, and scanning (e.g., feeling keyed up or on edge all the time).

Panic disorder is characterized by recurrent panic attacks, which are discrete periods of apprehension or fear accompanied by such symptoms as dyspnea, palpitations, choking, chest pain or discomfort, sweating, dizziness, fear of going crazy, and uncontrolled behavior. The first panic attack usually occurs in the patient's early 20s and appears unexpectedly. Many panic disorder patients develop severe phobic avoidance (agoraphobia). Such patients are not likely to be able to participate in an exercise class or program, although doing so would be of great benefit. Chronic anxiety can occur secondary to psychiatric problems besides depression, such as alcoholism, drug abuse, and schizophrenia. It can also be caused by medical problems, most commonly hyperthyroidism,

hypoglycemia, and temporal lobe epilepsy (Taylor & Arnow, 1988). Cardiovascular symptoms, particularly palpitations, are common in panic disorder patients
and many such patients first go to cardiologists believing they have heart disease.
As many as 30% of patients with normal coronary arteries on angiography
experience panic attacks, with about as many women as men falling into this
category.

Panic disorder is a very treatable condition, but the diagnosis must be made.
Consider enlisting the help of professionals who specialize in treating the problem
who will help the patient use an exercise program for psychological treatment.

Helping Patients With Anxiety

Some patients with anxiety report unpleasant symptoms when exercising. Use
of a treadmill can help reassure anxious patients that exercise is safe, and can
help the exercise instructor identify any contraindications to exercise (Taylor &
Houston Miller, 1993). Furthermore, exercise may help reduce symptoms in
patients with severe anxiety disorders.

Alcohol and Drug Abuse

Alcohol abuse is very common, occurring in at least 5 to 10% of the adult U.S.
population. Alcohol can impair judgment and memory, and in higher doses
is cardiotoxic and increases cardiovascular morbidity and mortality (Klatsky,
Armstrong, & Friedman, 1992). Alcohol abuse, besides being dangerous in itself,
significantly affects the success of lifestyle change programs. Alcoholism and
smoking are co-morbid conditions: as many as 10% of smokers are alcoholic,
and over 80% of alcoholics are smokers. Alcohol use is therefore a common
cause of relapse following smoking cessation.

Helping Patients With Alcohol Problems

When a health care professional has identified an individual as having a potential
alcohol problem on the basis of the CAGE or other information, he or she should
openly discuss the issue with the patient and provide referral to an alcohol
treatment program if appropriate. Alcoholism is treatable, and cardiac rehabilitation professionals can contribute significantly to a patients' overall well-being
by identifying alcoholism and making the appropriate referral. For information
on treatment programs for alcohol and other drug problems, consult the telephone
book's Yellow Pages under ''Alcoholism Information'' or ''Drug Abuse and
Addiction Information.'' Especially helpful is the Council on Alcoholism (or
Council on Alcohol and Drug Abuse), which can provide information about
nearby alcohol treatment programs. Alcoholics Anonymous (AA) and Narcotics
Anonymous (NA) also offer help for people with alcohol or drug problems. The
National Clearinghouse for Alcohol and Drug Information (1-800-729-6686) can
also provide the telephone numbers of local or state alcohol treatment programs.

Confronting the alcoholic patient is difficult for most health care professionals, and most alcoholic patients resist efforts to make them give up drinking. However, confrontation is essential if the patient is to overcome denial. Equivocal messages are likely to be ignored. It is preferable to say: "Based on these facts (provide appropriate information from CAGE, clinical interviews, reported consumption, medical examination, etc.), I believe you suffer from alcohol dependence and I would like to refer you for treatment."

Inadequate Social Support

Social support is a complicated phenomenon and researchers argue about how best to measure it. However, a few simple questions may provide the most important information. Those who never married or who live alone, and those who are less socially connected with a group or spouse, have a higher risk of heart disease and of overall mortality than do the socially connected (Case, Moss, Case, McDermott, & Eberly, 1992; Ruberman et al., 1984; Williams et al., 1992). For example, Ruberman et al. (1984) found that high-stressed, post-MI men had more than four times the mortality rate of socially involved, low-stressed, post-MI men. Socially isolated, post-MI women may have an even higher risk of recurrent major cardiac events than men (Case et al., 1992). For older patients, the loss of a loved one is associated with increased risk for all causes of mortality, and women, due to their greater longevity, are especially likely to experience the death of a loved one.

We do not know how social isolation affects morbidity and mortality. It may be that socially isolated individuals have less access to medical resources, pursue a less healthy lifestyle, are less willing to act on symptoms requiring medical attention, or are in a more dangerous physiological state. Patients who fall into one of the following categories may need extra help in overcoming the effects of social isolation:

a. Patients who live alone

b. Patients who have recently lost a loved one

c. Patients who feel socially isolated or alone or are very dissatisfied with their level of social support

Helping Patients With Inadequate Social Support

Rehabilitation programs can contribute to a patient's quality of life by providing social support. Several studies have demonstrated that telephone contact facilitates care and may even reduce mortality, especially when it involves monitoring the patient's stress level (Frasure-Smith & Prince, 1985). Participation in group programs undoubtedly has similar effects, particularly if at least some attention is given to interactive, social activities. Socially isolated individuals often benefit from a referral to a support group or from psychotherapy.

On the other hand, socially isolated individuals may need more and/or a different type of social contact than is normally available to them. Such individuals may make excessive demands on the staff of a rehabilitation program. In the MULTIFIT program, nurses often want to help such patients, yet dread phone calls that seem to go on endlessly. When such a patient begins to require too much time and effort, it can be a sign that he or she should be referred to a more appropriate program. At times, health care professionals must be quite firm, making it very clear that there are limits on the time available to each patient.

Handouts, videotapes, books, and other self-help materials can be useful to address certain kinds of problems, such as family functioning. We developed a simple two-page handout which briefly discusses family issues affected by the MI (see "MULTIFIT Information for Spouses," p. 40). The handout is given to the family members and they are encouraged to read it. Further clarification, elaboration, and referral are provided as needed.

There are many other psychosocial issues facing caridac patients: sex, intimacy, the return to work, changes in self-esteem, and family dynamics are all significant matters. The five factors discussed in detail here are not the only important ones, but their impact on multifactorial risk reduction is clear.

Summary

Many aspects of psychological functioning affect a patient's ability to make lifestyle changes. By using simple tools to screen for depression, anxiety, alcohol and drug abuse, social isolation, stress, and anger, the health care professional can identify problems requiring individualized education and support.

Psychosocial Questionnaire

Name _____ Date _____

For the first four questions, please circle a number on the scale following each item to show how much you are troubled now by each emotion.

1. Feeling miserable or depressed

1	2	3	4	5	6	7	8	9

Hardly   Slightly   Moderately   Markedly   Very severely

2. Feeling irritable or angry

1	2	3	4	5	6	7	8	9

Hardly   Slightly   Moderately   Markedly   Very severely

3. Feeling tense, anxious, or panicky

1	2	3	4	5	6	7	8	9

Hardly   Slightly   Moderately   Markedly   Very severely

4. Feeling under stress or pressure at work or at home

1	2	3	4	5	6	7	8	9

Hardly   Slightly   Moderately   Markedly   Very severely

5. Would you like help with any of these areas?

Depression   No ___ Yes ___   Anxiety   No ___ Yes ___
Anger   No ___ Yes ___   Stress   No ___ Yes ___

6. Do you ever drink alcohol?

___ No (go to #13)

___ Yes

	No	Yes

7. Have you ever felt you ought to cut down on your drinking?   ___ ___

8. Have people ever annoyed you by criticizing your drinking?   ___ ___

9. Have you ever felt bad or guilty about your drinking?   ___ ___

10. Have you ever had a drink first thing in the morning ("eye ___ ___
opener") to steady your nerves or get rid of a hangover?

11. About how often do you drink alcohol?

1   Daily or almost every day

2   3 or 4 times per week

3   Once or twice per week

4   Once or twice per month

5   Less often than once per month

6   Never

12. How many of these alcoholic beverages do you drink during an average
WEEK?

___ # of 12-oz bottles or cans of beer, ale, etc.

___ # of 4-oz glasses of wine, sherry, port, etc.

___ # of shots (one shot = 1.5 oz) of vodka, rum, scotch, whiskey, bourbon,
tequila, or gin (including mixed drinks and cocktails)

___ # of after-dinner drinks or liqueurs

13. Do you live alone?

___ No

___ Yes

14. Who helps you at home? _____

Thank you for your responses to these questions. This information will remain
confidential.

MULTIFIT Information for Spouses

Husbands

This information addresses common concerns of husbands of women who have had a heart attack. A heart attack is a crisis that affects your entire family and can trigger many emotions. As with any crisis, many people feel shock or disbelief, fear, anger, guilt, and sadness. These feelings are very normal and will probably go away in 4 to 6 weeks. Being aware of your feelings and discussing them with your wife and family members are important parts of dealing with the crisis of a heart attack. Talking to a trusted friend may also help to lessen your fears and anxieties. If after 4 to 6 weeks you are still having a difficult time working through these issues, you should think about seeking help from a health care professional such as your doctor, a nurse, or a therapist.

There are several common reactions and concerns among men whose spouses have had a heart attack. These issues, and recommendations for handling them, are listed below.

1. **Feelings of guilt.** It is natural to feel guilty. Many husbands are afraid they may have caused or contributed to the heart attack. A husband's common reaction is, "Perhaps she carried the burden of our family."

   Recommendation: Remember that many factors cause coronary heart disease and that it is highly unlikely that just stress or diet or smoking caused an attack. Rather than dwelling on the causes of the heart attack, think about ways you can reduce future risks. For example, learn how to help your wife manage stress, if necessary, instead of dwelling on the past. (See #5 for more suggestions.)

2. **Fear of being widowed.** It is not unusual, in the early stages of recovery, to fear losing one's wife or to feel isolated.

   Recommendation: Talk to your spouse and other family members about such fears; it may help to ease them. Often, your spouse has the same fears. Topics such as finances, insurance policies, property, and preparation of wills are difficult to discuss, but it is important to face them in the event of a life-threatening situation. Some husbands worry that such a discussion may cause stress; however, addressing such concerns may make your wife feel relieved and more prepared for the future.

3. **Household management.** Increased responsibility for managing the family is often an overwhelming burden for spouses in the early stages of recovery.

   Recommendation: Don't be afraid to ask for help. In a time of crisis, such as a heart attack, many friends and relatives feel helpless too and may want to help. Allowing others to provide meals, take turns at the hospital, or watch the children may be most helpful to your own well-being. Also, don't be afraid to set limits—especially on visitors and phone calls.

4. **Sexual relations.** Returning to a normal sex life may be difficult for both you and your wife. Often one or both partners experience a lack of drive or interest, and the husband may worry about whether sex is safe for his wife.

Recommendation: Although it may be difficult, make sure your wife's physician discusses this subject with both you and her before hospital discharge. Don't be afraid to talk to one another about your concerns. Start slowly. Other forms of lovemaking, such as kissing and holding, may be needed as an intermediate step before resuming sexual intercourse. If sexual problems become an issue, seek help by discussing these with your physician.

5. **Support for your wife.** The most difficult challenge for husbands is knowing how to be supportive of their wives after a heart attack. Husbands whose wives were responsible for many of the household chores may have difficulty responding to new demands. In addition, husbands often feel unprepared for the lifestyle changes their wives need to make.

Recommendation: Although being supportive means different things in different marriages, there are some general steps you can take to support your wife without being overprotective.

General Ways to Be Supportive and Help Yourself

- Don't be afraid to ask questions of all health care workers, especially the doctor. You and your wife need the same information to cooperate in her recovery.
- Reduce your stress at home by setting aside time for you and your spouse to talk or be together quietly. Communicate openly about your fears, anxieties, and needs.
- Comment on positive changes. Praise your wife's accomplishments, such as quitting smoking, exercising regularly, and changing eating habits.
- Beware of reminding. Reminding is often thought of as nagging or criticism. Research shows that this does not help people change and often makes people angry. Instead, be there to congratulate your spouse when she successfully takes small steps.
- Constantly remind yourself that you are not responsible for your spouse's health. She needs to take responsibility herself.

You can be most supportive by: (a) being prepared for a change in your wife's symptoms and (b) helping with lifestyle changes when you can. Use the tips below to help you.

Preparing for a Change in Symptoms

- Make sure you have the physician's telephone number(s) posted where all household members can see it. Talk about a plan for calling for help if symptoms of a serious problem occur.
- Ask your wife—**but not often**—if she is having any chest discomfort.
- Make sure extra nitroglycerin is kept in the original dark bottle and replace it every 6 months to 1 year. Allow your wife to take responsibility for carrying nitroglycerin.
- Know the warning signs of another heart attack.
- Take a cardio-pulmonary resuscitation (CPR) class offered through the YMCA or Red Cross. Refresh your skills every year.

Helping With Dietary Changes

- Continue eating out or dining with friends. Discuss with your wife how to do so without sacrificing a healthy diet.
- Don't worry about an occasional splurge. Remember, a treat on special occasions, such as birthdays or Thanksgiving, is healthy for one's attitude.
- Try to make **gradual** changes in eating habits. Avoid drastic limitations of food items. Slow changes will often be better maintained.
- Take a shopping trip to the grocery store together. Read labels and select foods appealing to both of you.

Starting an Exercise Program

- Think about exercising together. If your wife is able, walking 20 to 30 minutes per day will be helpful for you both.
- Suggest recreational activities and short trips that involve walking or other forms of physical activity (a trip to the mall, a short hike, etc.).
- Ask your spouse if she would like to be reminded to exercise once or twice a week.
- Help your wife to be more active when you are out together by parking farther away from shops, walking up flights of stairs instead of taking elevators, etc.

Helping With Smoking Cessation

- Make sure all ashtrays and cigarettes are removed from the house before your wife comes home from the hospital.
- If you smoke and find it difficult to quit now, promise yourself to do the following: Don't offer your wife cigarettes, keep cigarettes out of sight so your wife isn't tempted, and smoke outside the house as much as possible. Ask other family members who smoke to do the same.
- Praise your wife for not smoking.

We hope that the above suggestions are helpful as you go through this recovery process. We believe that your recovery is as important as your wife's. Take time to be aware of your feelings, to voice your concerns, to get answers to your questions, and to take care of yourself.

Wives

This information addresses common concerns of wives of men who have had a heart attack. A heart attack is a crisis that affects your entire family and can trigger many emotions. As with any crisis, many people feel shock or disbelief, fear, anger, guilt, and sadness. These feelings are very normal and will probably go away in 4 to 6 weeks. Being aware of your feelings and discussing them with your husband and family members are important parts of dealing with the crisis of a heart attack. Talking to a trusted friend may also help to lessen your fears and anxieties. If after 4 to 6 weeks you are still having a difficult time working through these issues, you should think about seeking help from a health care professional such as your doctor, a nurse, or a therapist.

We know there are common reactions and concerns among women whose husbands have had a heart attack. These issues and recommendations for handling them are listed below.

1. **Feelings of guilt.** It is natural to feel guilty. Many wives are afraid they may have caused or contributed to the heart attack. A wife's common reaction is, ''I caused the heart attack because of the food I served.''

   Recommendation: Remember that many factors cause coronary heart disease and it is highly unlikely that just diet or stress or smoking caused an attack. Rather than dwelling on the causes of the heart attack, think about ways you can reduce future risks. For example, learn how to change your family's eating habits rather than worrying about past eating patterns. Under number 7 below you'll find more suggestions.

2. **Fear of widowhood.** It is not unusual in the early stages of recovery, and wives tend to feel isolated.

   Recommendation: Talk to your spouse and other family members about such fears; it may help to ease them. Often your spouse has the same fears. Topics such as finances, insurance policies, property, and preparation of wills are difficult to discuss, but are important in the face of any major crisis. Some wives worry that such a discussion may cause stress; however, your husband may be relieved and feel more prepared for the future.

3. **Household management.** Increased responsibility for managing the family is often an overwhelming burden for spouses in the early stages of recovery.

   Recommendation: Don't be afraid to ask for help. In a time of crisis such as a heart attack, many friends and relatives feel helpless too and may want to help. Allowing others to provide meals, take turns at the hospital, or watch the children may be most helpful to your own well-being. Also, don't be afraid to set limits—especially on visitors and phone calls.

4. **Anxiety and depression.** Many wives experience anxiety, fear, and depression. These feelings usually result in sleeplessness, upset stomach, and lack of energy. Some wives may also become short tempered with spouse, family, and friends.

Recommendation: Feeling anxious and depressed is a normal response to the crisis. Anxiety and depression often go away after 3 to 4 weeks. You'll feel less anxious if you know what to expect when your husband gets home, when he can return to normal activities, and how you can help change risk factors. Ask your physician and nurse for this information. If you still feel anxious or depressed after a month, consider getting professional help.

5. **Personal time.** Sometimes wives are so involved in their husband's recovery that they find they have no time for themselves.

Recommendation: Realize you are important, and take time for yourself— even 15 to 30 minutes per day. Do things that please you, such as working on a favorite hobby, gardening, shopping, or reading. You'll be better prepared to handle stress if you concentrate on your needs too. If you are employed, consider returning to work as soon as possible. Work can distract you and may be a reward.

6. **Sexual relations.** Returning to a normal sex life may be difficult for both you and your husband. Often there is a lack of drive or interest for one partner or both, and concerns about whether it is safe for your husband.

Recommendation: Although it may be difficult, make sure your husband's physician discusses this subject with you both before hospital discharge. Don't be afraid to talk to one another about your concerns. Start slowly. Other forms of lovemaking such as kissing and holding may be an initial step toward resuming sexual intercourse. If sexual problems become an issue, seek help by discussing these with your physician.

7. **Support for your husband.** The hardest thing for wives is knowing how to be supportive of their husbands after a heart attack. Normally, wives become overprotective or overinvolved out of concern for their spouse's welfare. In addition, wives often feel unprepared for the lifestyle changes their husbands need to make.

Recommendation: Although being supportive means different things in different marriages, there are some general steps you can take to support your husband without being overprotective.

General Ways to Be Supportive and Help Yourself

- Don't be afraid to ask questions of all health care workers, especially the doctor. You and your husband need the same information to cooperate in his recovery.
- Reduce your stress at home by setting aside time for you and your spouse to talk or be together quietly. Communicate openly about your fears, anxieties, and needs.
- State the positive. Praise your husband's accomplishments such as quitting smoking, exercising regularly, and changing eating habits.
- Beware of reminding. Reminding is often thought of as nagging or criticism. Research shows that this does not help people change, and often makes people angry. Instead, be there to congratulate your spouse when small steps occur.
- Constantly remind yourself that you are not responsible for your husband's health. He needs to take responsibility himself.

You can be most supportive by (a) being prepared for a change in your husband's symptoms and (b) helping with lifestyle changes when you can. Use the tips below to help you.

Preparing for a Change in Symptoms

- Make sure you have the physician's telephone number(s) posted for all household members. Talk about a plan for calling for help if symptoms occur.
- Ask your husband—but not too often—if he is having any chest discomfort.
- Make sure extra nitroglycerin is kept in the refrigerator and replace it every 6 to12 months. Allow your husband to take responsibility for carrying nitroglycerin.
- Know the warning signs of another heart attack.
- Take a CPR class offered through the YMCA or Red Cross. Refresh your skills every year.

Helping With Dietary Changes

- Let go of the responsibility you feel for the things you can't control, such as meals and snacks away from home. Instead, work with your husband to develop a list of appropriate food choices for these times.
- Buy low-fat, low-cholesterol foods that you know your spouse will eat. Don't force your husband to eat foods that he doesn't enjoy.
- Continue eating out or dining with friends. Discuss with your husband how to do it healthfully.
- Don't worry about an occasional splurge. Remember, a treat on special occasions, such as birthdays or Thanksgiving, is healthy for one's attitude.
- Try to make gradual changes in eating habits. Avoid drastic limitations of food items. Slow changes will often be better maintained.

- Take a shopping trip to the grocery store together. Read labels and select foods appealing to both you and your spouse.
- Allow your husband to take part in meal planning and/or preparation at least one day per week.

Starting an Exercise Program

- Think about exercising together. If he is able, walking 20 to 30 minutes per day will be helpful for you both.
- Suggest recreational activities and short trips that involve walking or other forms of physical activity (e.g., a trip to the mall, a short hike).
- Ask your spouse if he would like to be reminded to exercise once or twice a week.
- Help your husband to be more active when you are out together (e.g., park farther away from shops, walk flights of stairs instead of taking elevators).

Helping With Smoking Cessation

- Make sure all ashtrays and cigarettes are removed from the house before your husband comes home from the hospital.
- If you smoke and find it difficult to quit now, promise yourself to do the following: Don't offer your husband cigarettes, keep cigarettes out of sight so your husband isn't tempted, and smoke outside the house as much as possible. Ask other family members who smoke to do the same.
- Praise your husband for not smoking.

We hope that the above suggestions are helpful as you go through this recovery process. We believe that your recovery is as important as your husband's. Take time to be aware of your feelings, to voice your concerns, to get answers to your questions, and to take care of yourself.

Chapter 5

Adherence
to Exercise Programs

E xercise is an important component of lifestyle change programs. Exercise training has been shown to have beneficial effects on lipid profiles (Hartung, Squires, & Gotto, 1981) and to lower both systolic and diastolic blood pressure in patients with mild to moderate hypertension (Hagberg, Montain, Martin, & Ehsani, 1989). Exercise can also have a positive impact on other health-related behaviors. For example, exercise in association with dietary modification can have a major effect on weight loss (Wood, Stefanick, Williams, & Haskell, 1991), it can help reduce the urge to smoke if applied as a technique for relapse prevention (Knapp, 1988), and it can serve as a useful stress reducing technique to help patients deal with the emotions of everyday life (Stern & Cleary, 1981). In North America there have been no clinical trials large enough to test the hypothesis that exercise can independently reduce subsequent morbidity and mortality from coronary heart disease. However, meta-analysis of 22 studies of post-MI patients in cardiac rehabilitation has shown a reduction of 25% in 1-year to 3-year rates of total cardiovascular events and total mortality, compared to control patients (May, Eberlein, Furberg, Passamani, & DeMets, 1982; O'Connor, Buring, & Yusaf, 1989; Oldridge, Guyalit, Fischer, & Rimm, 1988). In addition to reducing cardiovascular events, exercise may have a very strong impact on risk factors.

Of all of the health-related behaviors, exercise appears to be the most easily adopted behavior for patients with coronary heart disease. But the maintenance of this behavior is more problematic. Research beginning in the early 1980s indicates, for example, that roughly 50% of program participants will drop out of an exercise program during the first 12 months (Oldridge, 1982). In a more recent report, Oldridge (1991) found the rate of dropout from cardiac rehabilitation to be between 25 and 30% at 3 months, increasing to 40% at 6 months, and 50% at 12 months.

Because 85% of cardiac rehabilitation programs in the United States are hospital based (Thomas et al., in press), the initial 10 to 12 weeks of exercise training represents the adoption phase of this behavior. Most programs are limited to 12 weeks, and it is during this adoption period that education, counseling, and skills must be applied to ensure that the patient continues with the maintenance of the exercise behavior. In this chapter we discuss the reasons for nonadherence,

Table 5.1   Review of Exercise Adherence Studies (Home Training)

Study	Adherence strategies	Measurement of adherence	Adherence (% of prescribed sessions)		
			3 mos.	6 mos.	12 mos.
DeBusk et al. (1985) Post-MI patients (home vs. group)	Telephone calls Daily activity logs	Activity logs	89% (home) 84% (gym)	72% (home) 71% (gym)	—
Rogers et al. (1987) Sedentary, middle-aged men/ women (home)	Daily activity logs	Solid-state micro-compressor (Vitalog)	—	108% (male) 90% (female)	—
King et al. (1988) Community-based, middle-aged men/ women (home vs. group)	Daily activity logs, mailed monthly	Activity logs Self report			78.7% (high intensity home) 75.1% (low intensity home) 52.6% (gym)
DeBusk et al. (1994) Post-MI patients (home vs. usual care)	Daily activity logs (2-month) Monthly telephone calls (6 months)	Telephone follow-up of activity logs	—	72% (home) 58% (usual care)	71% (home) 55% (usual care)

outline intervention strategies for maintenance, and highlight key components contributing to patients' successful maintenance of exercise in home-based reha-bilitation. Table 5.1 summarizes findings from our studies concerning successful adherence to home exercise training.

Nonadherence to Exercise Programs

Reviews of the literature on nonadherence to exercise programs have often categorized contributing factors as personal, behavioral, and environmental or programmatic (King & Martin, 1993). Personal factors include

- age;
- body weight;
- smoking status;
- past experience with exercise;
- perception of one's health status;
- self-efficacy beliefs; and
- perceptions of access to facilities, availability of time, and exercise intensity.

Another personal factor which may effect adherence is self-motivation (Dishman & Steinhardt, 1988). Behavioral factors include

- the patient's skill and his or her ability to carry out exercise while minimizing injury and boredom, and
- impediments to exercise, such as travel.

Environmental and programmatic factors include

- lack of family support,
- proximity to exercise facilities,
- access to facilities if patients are involved in group programs,
- the flexibility of the exercise regimen,
- weather, and
- cues within the environment, such as reminders to exercise.

While all of these factors must be considered in working with patients to develop appropriate skills for exercise program maintenance, there are several factors which have been linked to a higher dropout rate and poor attendance in those who have participated in formal cardiac rehabilitation programs. These include smoking, blue-collar occupation, low socioeconomic status, obesity, angina pectoris, anxiety, depression, low self-motivation, poor social support, and the inconvenience of the location or timing of the program (Andrew, Oldridge, & Parker, 1981; Dishman & Gettman, 1980; Oldridge, 1982). Recent evidence also suggests that women under 45 years and on Medicaid may also be a population at high risk for dropout (Oldridge, Ragowski, & Gottleib, 1992).

Rehabilitation programs should include methods to identify patients who are likely to drop out. The easiest way to do this is simply to systematically and routinely ask patients how likely they are to begin exercising and, once they are exercising, how likely are they to continue to exercise. Interventions should be developed to deal with the patient's reasons for not wanting to exercise or wanting to drop out. The "Pre-Exercise Assessment Questionnaire" (p. 55) may be used to assess the level of committment to exercise of patients who are not already involved in a rehabilitation program. These questions should be administered in an interview conducted by a health care professional.

Intervention Strategies
for Maintenance of Exercise Programs

Various studies have shown that certain behavior strategies affect the likelihood that a patient will continue to exercise. Contracting, providing social support, relapse prevention techniques, and generalization training are such strategies.

Contracting

As with many other lifestyle changes, behavioral strategies have been successful for exercise adherence when implemented in healthy clinic and cardiac populations. Contracting, written agreements, and goal setting are examples of behavioral strategies which have proven effective in increasing patients' attendance (Oldridge & Jones, 1983). When using contracts or written agreements, however, it is important to ensure that the goals are well defined and that the contract specifies a renewal date. All too often, the patient is expected to attend three group exercise sessions per week, but there is no clear, written definition of a goal. As a very specific goal, it could be noted on a contract or written agreement that the patient is expected to attend at least 80% of all sessions during a given month. It might also be useful to use exercise attendance as a strategy to reach other goals, such as weight loss. When assessing patients' adherence to an exercise program, it is important to remember that many patients exercise on their own outside the program.

Social Support

Social support has been shown to increase adherence to exercise. As discussed in chapter 2, social support can be provided by spouses or family members, by health care professionals, or by friends, whose help can be enlisted by using a "buddy system." Spousal participation in exercise sessions has been found to be related to an increase in the frequency and duration of participation in Phase III cardiac rehabilitation sessions (Burkett, Rectanus, & Bultena, 1990). Once a patient is ready to leave the program, or if the patient is involved in home exercise, the goal should be to incorporate as many forms of social support as possible. These might include telephone calls from the program's director, newsletters, exercising with friends and coworkers, and praise by family members.

Self-Monitoring and Feedback

Self-monitoring and feedback may also enhance the patient's motivation to exercise. Daily activity logs such as the one shown on p. 56 provide the patient with important physiological data (heart rates, rating of perceived exertion [RPE], etc.) and may help the health care professional monitor the patient's development and changes in symptoms during the adoption phase of exercise. For home exercise training, we have found these logs to be invaluable in helping patients monitor their daily exercise sessions. For maintenance of exercise, a weekly activity log is more appropriate than a daily one. A sample "Weekly Exercise Activity Log" for early maintenance is shown on page 58. An "Exercise Plan and Tip Sheet" (p. 59), used in conjunction with the activity log, helps patients identify strategies for getting back on track if they should fail to exercise.

Feedback in the form of praise for exercising is most important as patients adopt an exercise behavior. Feedback can be provided by a health care professional in the early stages of exercise, but during the maintenance phase, if patients are not involved in a group program, they must rely upon other methods of feedback, such as praise from a spouse or family member. Other forms of feedback can also provide important incentives to maintain an exercise program. For many individuals, it is useful to undergo a repeat treadmill exercise test 3, 6, or 12 months after initiation of the exercise program. Motivation to continue exercise can also come from the patient's observing a change in his or her functional capacity; observing reduction in rate pressure product; and noticing a change in physiological feelings, such as decreases in fatigue and dyspnea.

Some patients may benefit from using self-administered exercise assessments to see improvement. Such tests allow patients to measure their current level of activity against their past performance and can provide positive feedback similar to obtaining a lower cholesterol level after a short course of dietary intervention. Figure 5.1 shows an example of the type of assessment we have used in order for patients to note their progress on a weekly basis. This graph could also be used to assess monthly improvement. Patients using this technique are asked to walk continually for 20 minutes while maintaining a given heart rate (normally 70 or 85% of the maximum heart rate on treadmill testing). At the end of the 20 minutes, they record the distance walked on the self-test chart. Distance can be measured with a car odometer. In succeeding weeks they perform the same self-test, using the same heart rate but noting any change in the distance walked. As patients become more fit, they are able to walk a longer distance in the same amount of time, thus providing feedback and further motivation. The chart is kept on the patient's refrigerator as a reminder to exercise.

Relapse Prevention

Relapse prevention training, most applicable to addictive behaviors, has some application to exercise, particularly when a patient lapses from a regular exercise schedule. The Abstinence Violation Effect of taking an initial cigarette or drink is a well-known problem for smokers and drinkers (a lapse that can lead to full-blown relapse), but no one has defined the time period after which a lapse from exercise leads to a total relapse. We believe the threat of total relapse exists when an individual misses more than a week of exercise that is regularly performed three to five times per week. The weekly self-monitoring log is designed to provide warning signals when such a threat exists, and to give patients suggestions for maintaining their programs if their exercise sessions begin to decline.

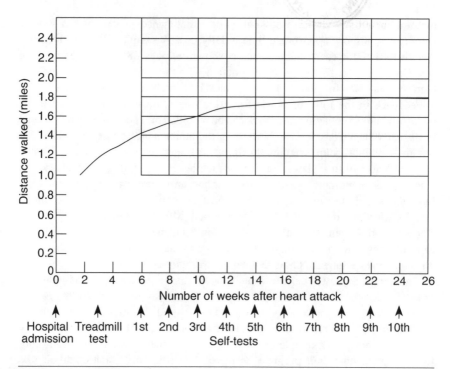

Figure 5.1   Self-test chart for walking: distance walked in 20 minutes. A sample plot for a patient exercising 3 to 4 times a week is shown on the chart.

Following the relapse prevention model, it is important to prepare individuals both psychologically and behaviorally for breaks or slips in their activity pattern. Individuals must be warned that such breaks are inevitable, and they must be taught to identify their own high-risk situations—those which can lead to full-blown relapse. High-risk situations causing patients to lapse from exercise include a break in a person's activity schedule due to an illness or injury, travel, bad weather conditions, increased demand at work, and boredom (Sallis, Haskell, & Fortmann, 1986). These high-risk situations can be assessed through the use of self-monitoring logs whereby patients keep track of the times they fail to exercise, or through self-efficacy ratings applied before initiation of an exercise program. Several recent studies have demonstrated that relapse prevention techniques in combination with other cognitive and behavioral strategies may improve long-term adherence to exercise, especially in middle-aged men and women (King et al., 1988; King & Frederiksen, 1984).

Generalization Training

For those people involved in formal cardiac rehabilitation programs, it is important to incorporate what behaviorists term "generalization training" into a plan for maintenance of exercise. Generalization means that the behavior is generalized from a specific situation (where it was initiated) to a variety of situations. Generalization training prepares an individual for transition from a group program to nongroup, and usually, outside activities. (King & Martin, 1993). To ensure the patient's adherence to exercise at home, generalization training can be accomplished by asking a patient to exercise in an unsupervised environment beginning one to two times per week before leaving the program; having family members attend formal exercise sessions to provide support and feedback before the patient leaves the program; and incorporating various forms of exercise into the regimen that an individual is likely to undertake at home (King & Martin, 1993). In some instances, gradually decreasing the number of formal sessions a patient is expected to attend may also be appropriate. Other behavioral techniques, such as instruction, feedback/praise, and self-monitoring of attendance, must be taken over by the patient.

Home Training—The MULTIFIT Experience

During the past 15 years, our experience in providing strategies to help patients maintain their exercise training at home has resulted in high adherence rates to exercise one year after program initiation. Further studies are needed to confirm the longer-term rates of adherence following participation in both supervised programs and home programs, but the strategies employed in this program may help to explain the adherence rate of 71% at one year, in the 85% of all post-MI patients eligible to participate in the home training program within MULTIFIT (DeBusk et al., 1994). Patients continue to report exercising on average five times per week for a total of 34 ± 18 minutes per session at 12 months following their event.

The components of the MULTIFIT Exercise Training Program are noted below.

IN HOSPITAL

- Written "Early Activity" guidelines
- Active Partnership™ video and workbook on exercise
- Education about pulse-checking/heart-rate guidelines

OUTPATIENT

- Symptom-limited treadmill test 3 to 4 weeks after MI/CABG
- Written guidelines for home exercise
- Exer-Sentry™ heart rate monitors (first 8 weeks)
- Daily activity logs (first 8 weeks)
- Monthly telephone calls by nurse (6 months)
- Monthly activity logs (first 9 months)
- Self-tests for assessing improvement (as needed)

In the MULTIFIT Program, patients are provided a one-page handout that prepares them to begin a walking program upon discharge. They view the Active

Partnership™ videotape in hospital, if time permits, or at home, and are instructed on how to monitor their heart rates. After the patient completes a symptom-limited treadmill test (normally around 18 to 21 days post-infarction), he or she takes part in a 15- to 20-minute counseling session on exercise, conducted by the nurse. At this session, patients are provided written guidelines for home exercise. They are asked to exercise for 30 minutes per day, 5 days per week, and are allowed to choose the form of aerobic exercise (often alternating between two activities to ensure increased adherence and enjoyability). In the MULTIFIT Program, 72% of patients chose walking as their main form of exercise. Patients are asked to use heart rate monitors for a period of 8 weeks in order to increase their adherence to the program and help them regulate exercise intensity. They are also taught how to use rating of perceived exertion (RPE) as another method of monitoring exercise intensity.

Patients follow daily exercise sessions for a period of 8 weeks and use daily activity logs (shown on p. 56) to record each session. These are mailed back to the nurse every 2 weeks and incorporated as part of a structured telephone call. After 8 weeks, patients move to weekly monitoring logs (shown on p. 58). Monthly telephone calls directed at all risk factors supplement adherence strategies. The portion of the call related to exercise focuses on questions about the intensity of training, symptoms, and barriers to adherence. In the 10-minute call, the nurse provides positive reinforcement for continued performance, helps the patient address difficulties he or she may be having with prescriptions or adherence to exercise, and seeks to detect any changes in symptoms that would warrant contact with the primary care physician. After 6 months, patients return for follow-up treadmill testing and the maintenance phase of the program begins. They reaffirm their committment to exercise, assess potential high-risk situations that could lead to a lapse in exercise, and continue to monitor their weekly adherence. If they lapse after 2 to 3 weeks, they are instructed to call their nurse for help. After 9 months, one structured telephone call by the nurse encourages the patient to continue the program and helps him or her with difficulties in adhering to the regimen. By this time, most patients have incorporated into their daily routines their own self-management strategies for exercise.

Summary

While not all patients can undertake exercise training following a coronary heart disease event, the vast majority are eligible to perform aerobic exercise. A planned approach to helping patients maintain their exercise program is critical during the early stages of adoption. Adherence strategies such as contracting, self-monitoring, feedback, and relapse prevention may increase the likelihood that a patient will be successful in maintaining the exercise program.

Pre-Exercise Assessment Questionnaire

1. Have you ever been involved in a structured exercise program? (Probe)

2. What has been your level of physical activity over the past year?

3. What is your perception of your health at the present time?

0	1	2	3
Poor	Fair	Good	Excellent

4. Do you disagree or agree with the following statement:
   "Exercise has little benefit to my overall health."

0	1	2	3	4
Strongly disagree	Disagree	Neither agree nor disagree	Agree	Strongly agree

5. What is your confidence in your ability to exercise 20 to 30 minutes, 3 times per week, over the next month?

0	10	20	30	40	50	60	70	80	90	100
No confidence					Fairly confident				Very confident	

6. Have you ever had success in engaging in leisure time physical activities? (Probe)

7. Are your spouse and other family members supportive of your taking time to exercise? Are they interested in exercising with you?

8. Will scheduling exercise or traveling to an exercise facility be problematic for you?

9. How likely are you to begin to exercise 20 to 30 minutes, 3 times per week, over the next month?

0	1	2	3	4
Not at all likely	Not very likely	Somewhat likely	Very likely	Very, very likely

Questions 3, 4, 5, and 9 ask patients to respond using scales. The scales should be read to patients when each question is asked.

MULTIFIT Daily Exercise Log

Name _____ For the 2-week period beginning _____

Target heart rate range ____ to ____ beats/min

_____ to ____ beats/10 sec

Rating of perceived exertion (RPE) ____ to ____
(See RPE scale)

Every time you exercise, record the following information in the space below:

- Date of exercise session
- Type of activity: W = walk, W-J = walk/jog,
  J = jog, B = bicycle, S = swim
- Length of time spent exercising in minutes
- Peak heart rate achieved
- Peak RPE achieved
- Comments: change in symptoms, lack of exer-
  cise, etc.

RPE Scale	
6	
7	Very, very light
8	
9	Very light
10	
11	Fairly light
12	
13	Somewhat hard
14	
15	Hard
16	
17	Very hard
18	
19	Very, very hard

Week 1:

	Example	Day 1	Day 2	Day 3	Day 4	Day 5	Day 6	Day 7
Date	5/26/92							
Activity	W							
Minutes	30 min							
Peak HR	110							
Peak RPE	13							
Symptoms	0							

Comments: _____

Week 2:

	Example	Day 1	Day 2	Day 3	Day 4	Day 5	Day 6	Day 7
Date	6/3/92							
Activity	W							
Minutes	30 min							
Peak HR	110							
Peak RPE	13							
Symptoms	0							

Comments: _____

Key to Symptoms: 0 = None   4 = Leg cramps
                   1 = Angina   5 = Nausea
                   2 = Shortness of breath   6 = Irregular heartbeats
                   3 = Dizziness   7 = Excessive fatigue

Weekly Exercise Activity Log

Name _____ Log # <u>1</u> 2   3   4   5   6

Date _____   (circle one)

Exercise

At the end of each week, **circle** the number of times you exercised that week. Then follow the instructions to the right.

Your target heart rate range is ____ beats/min to ____ beats/min.

Example	__ /__ /__	__ /__ /__	__ /__ /__	__ /__ /__
4+	4+	4+	4+	4+
③	3	3	3	3
2	2	2	2	2
1	1	1	1	1
0	0	0	0	0
	Ex. Week 1	Ex. Week 2	Ex. Week 3	Ex. Week 4

If you circled

   4+: Keep up the good work!

     3: See your Tip Sheet after 2 weeks at this level.

  1-2: See your Tip Sheet whenever you're in this range.

     0: Call for help now.

Comments: _____

_____

_____

_____

Exercise Plan and Tip Sheet

What's the Problem? I have exercised less or not at all this past week because of:

- ☐ Travel
- ☐ Vacation
- ☐ Crisis situation
- ☐ Illness or injury*

- ☐ Boredom with the exercise program
- ☐ Work pressures or schedule
- ☐ Other: _____

Make Your Plan. How can you alter, avoid, or adapt to this problem situation? Select two or three strategies from the tips below, or develop your own. Write your plan here and sign it with a person who can help.

During the next week I will

_____

_____

_____

_____

Your signature

_____

Signature of support person

Tips to Help You Get Back on Track

- Record your daily exercise sessions on a calendar.
- Monitor your performance by undertaking your self-test twice next week.
- Carry your exercise clothes in the car.
- Place your exercise clothes on your nightstand, where you'll see them.
- Ask a buddy to exercise with you for a week or two.
- Divide your daily exercise session into two 15-minute periods.
- Post a large sign in a visible spot reminding you to exercise. Put it on your refrigerator, telephone, front door, etc.
- Alternate between two activities during the next week or two.
- Try a new form of exercise to relieve boredom.
- Ask a family member to remind you to exercise 4 or 5 times next week.
- Try to exercise during the noon hour once or twice in the week.
- Think of a simple reward for yourself if you exercise 4 to 5 times next week.
- Be sure to take along exercise clothes when traveling.
- In times of crisis or unusual pressure, it is hard to stick to a schedule. Instead, ask yourself throughout the day if it would help to take a break for exercise.

*NOTE: These plans may not be appropriate during times of serious illness or injury. You can call your nurse for advice.

Chapter 6

Dietary Assessment and Intervention

Mia Clark, RD, MPH

L owering blood cholesterol levels with diet or drugs has been shown to decrease the incidence of coronary heart disease. A report on diet and health from the National Research Council, Committee on Diet and Health (1989) cites the many studies supporting this link. The association is strongest in middle-aged men with high serum cholesterol, but also holds for younger and older men, women, and patients with moderately elevated cholesterol. In addition, there is increasing evidence that reducing serum cholesterol through diet or drugs can contribute to the regression of coronary lesions (LaRosa et al., 1990). The relationship between elevated triglycerides and risk for CHD is less clear, except when associated with other dyslipidemias.

Persuasive data from animal, epidemiological, and clinical studies supports a causal relationship between diet (specifically high saturated fat and cholesterol intakes, and excessive caloric intake leading to obesity) and arteriosclerotic cardiovascular disease (National Diet-Heart Study Research Group, 1968). As a result of the Coronary Primary Prevention Trial (The Lipid Research Clinic, 1984) and the Framingham Study (Kannel, Castelli, Gordon, & McNamara, 1971), it is recognized that a 1% lowering in an individual's total serum cholesterol level results in a 2% (or greater) lowering in CHD risk. The expected plasma total cholesterol reduction is approximately 10 to 20% when dietary intake of saturated fat is decreased from 13% to less than 7% of calories and intake of cholesterol is reduced from 400-500 mg to less than 200 mg per day (Kris-Etherton et al., 1988). Plasma cholesterol changes may be less when the baseline diet contains only moderate amounts of saturated fat and cholesterol.

We know that excess body weight is positively correlated with blood cholesterol and blood pressure, and that weight loss can help reduce risk in relation to blood cholesterol, blood pressure, and diabetes (Jeffery, 1988). Benefits are evident following a loss of as little as a 4.5 kg (10 lb), even when this loss does not bring the patient down to ideal body weight.

Dietary Management: What the Nondietitian Can Do

A trained dietitian is the ideal source for dietary advice and counseling. However, cardiac patients typically see a dietitian once or twice, while seeing the doctor, nurse, or rehabilitation staff repeatedly over a longer period of time. For this reason, doctors, nurses, and other health care professionals should be prepared to provide primary counseling and support for dietary management. Unfortunately, many health care professionals feel insecure in this role. This chapter provides background information to help the health care professional become a more effective agent for dietary change. The chapter also provides the dietitian with some strategies that facilitate follow-up by other members of the patient's health care team.

The dietary recommendations that nondietitians can reinforce are summarized below. They are explained in detail in the pages that follow.

- Replace high-fat foods like meats, whole-fat dairy products, fried foods, and convenience foods with lower fat items like poultry and fish, fresh fruits and vegetables, breads and grains.
- Read food labels to find products with acceptable levels of fat.
- Follow a regular exercise program.
- Overweight patients should lose 4.5 kg (10 lb). A low-fat diet and regular exercise facilitate the achievement of this goal.
- Patients with elevated triglycerides (> 200 mg/dl) should restrict alcohol in addition to increasing exercise and reducing excess body weight.

General Considerations in Dietary Management

There are two very important ways in which dietary management differs from the management of other lifestyle patterns. First, diet involves choosing from among many possible options. Second, these choices must be made many times each day. These characteristics can overwhelm both patient and provider if they are not addressed early in the behavior change process.

A person eating three meals per day probably consumes at least two dozen distinct foods each day. If we include beverages and snack items, the total could rise by an additional dozen items. From one day to the next, some of the food items remain the same, and some new ones are introduced. In a week's time, an individual might consume as many as a hundred different edible items. Seasonal variations can result in further adjustments to the "weekly 100," and this may happen two or three times in a year. Indeed, dietitians encourage this type of dietary diversity because it helps ensure that the body's long-term nutritional needs are met.

To complicate matters further, a typical grocery store offers thousands of food choices. Different stores offer slightly different arrays of food items and brand names. Manufacturers constantly introduce new items and reformulate, repackage, and replace the existing ones. In light of such diversity and flux, dietary management can appear to be a daunting task for both the patient and the health care professional. In reality, however, there are certain natural boundaries to dietary patterns. Personal preferences limit the field of choices for any individual. Cultural and environmental factors (such as food availability) reduce this field still further.

The fact is that most people eat a fairly limited set of foods regularly, and another set of foods only occasionally.

The first step in dietary management is to determine which foods are preferred and eaten regularly and which, if any, are unacceptable. Then the health care professional and the patient can select a variety of foods to come up with a diet that is acceptable to the patient over the long term—or for the rest of his or her life!

Measuring Dietary Intake

There are many methods and tools for assessing the dietary intake of individuals and populations. However, it is an area lacking data with strict validity and reliability, largely because there is no absolute truth or "gold standard" by which tools can be tested (Rhoads, 1987). Diet is a behavior that defies objective, unobtrusive monitoring on a large scale. In addition, there are no clear physiological standards to which dietary measures can be compared. As a result, dietary assessment tools have been developed to approximate actual intake, as determined by the face validity of the tool and by its performance compared with the most widely accepted of the other assessment tools. Block (1982) has suggested that the results of dietary assessment be regarded as rankings on a scale of "high" to "low," rather than as absolute nutrient intake levels.

Measuring dietary intake in a free-living population requires us to rely on self-reported data, which are subject to errors in both perception and recall. Even food records (daily diaries kept by the patient) are subject to omissions and misperceptions. The very act of keeping records tends to influence what is eaten. Furthermore, self-reported dietary data consistently underestimates caloric intake, and thus the intake of macro-nutrients (carbohydrates, proteins, and fat). Still, self-report of dietary intake at periodic intervals is an important aspect of patient care because it provides the basis for a relevant discussion concerning dietary change. Multiple and repeated measures can give a fairly reliable picture of eating patterns and changes over time.

The four most commonly used tools for collecting individual dietary intake information are diet histories, food records, 24-hour recalls, and food frequency questionnaires. Food records are completed prospectively; histories, recalls, and frequencies are retrospective. Each tool has advantages and disadvantages that influence its appropriateness in different settings and programs.

Diet History

The diet history involves an extensive interview by a trained dietitian to determine the long-term dietary patterns of an individual. This method of dietary assessment has been used successfully in studies since the 1940s. The interview generally requires at least an hour to complete, and additional time is needed for analysis by the dietitian. Because the focus of the diet history is the patient's typical eating patterns over past years, it is not well suited for assessing recent or pending changes in diet.

Food Records

Food records are diaries that record the types and quantities of all foods and beverages consumed over a specified time period. Patients may be asked to estimate quantities or to measure them. Records are kept for three to seven days, including at least one weekend day. Food records usually provide more precise dietary information than the other methods, making them useful for detailed nutrient analysis. However, food records are tedious for the patient to keep and require sophisticated analysis in order to extract nutrient-specific data. Training patients to keep sufficiently detailed records can be burdensome also. Although food records are often considered the "gold standard" of dietary assessments, supporting validity and reliability data are incomplete.

24-Hour Recall

The 24-hour recall is a recounting of all foods and beverages consumed in a recent 24-hour period, usually the day—midnight to midnight—prior to the one on which the recall is taken. Patients estimate quantities for each item that was consumed. Recalls are typically taken in an office visit or during a telephone call from the health professional. The accuracy of recalls is limited by the patient's memory of details that are ordinarily ignored, such as exactly what was in the casserole and how many pretzels were eaten. Even when the patient's memory is excellent, a single 24-hour period is not considered representative of overall intake patterns, and therefore is not adequate for nutrient assessment of individual patients. However, the tool is quite acceptable for determining the intake of groups and subpopulations of individuals. Health care professionals often use the 24-hour recall with individual patients to look at certain dietary patterns like frequency of meals and snacks, variety of foods eaten in a day, and relative quantities of foods.

Food Frequency Questionnaires

Food frequency questionnaires list a number of food items, and patients indicate how often they eat each one. Responses are usually given in numbers of servings per day, per week, or per month, depending on the particular questionnaire being used. Food frequency questionnaires vary in the number of items listed and in the degree of specificity regarding quantities. The advantage of the food frequency method is that it provides a view of the bigger picture, as opposed to a particular day or week, and it allows us to determine which foods are eaten routinely and which ones are not. Frequency information, however, cannot be considered comprehensive, for it reflects only those foods listed on the questionnaire. Nutrient intake can be estimated from frequency data, but it cannot be calculated precisely.

For long-term management of the cardiac patient, repeated use of either food records or food frequency questionnaires is appropriate. Which method is used will depend largely on the institutional resources and skills available. For an institution that is already equipped with the staff and the technology to train patients to keep records and has the means to analyze the records to determine which foods contribute the most saturated fat and cholesterol, food records may be a good method to adopt. Otherwise, food frequency questionnaires are recommended for ease of completion and interpretation.

Several food frequency questionnaires have been developed and tested, and they have produced good results with respect to detecting dietary fat, saturated fat, and cholesterol intake. One such instrument is the "Food Frequency Questionnaire" (FFQ) which was developed for the MULTIFIT program. Sample FFQ items are shown on pages 73-74. The questionnaire consists of 43 items and takes approximately 10 minutes to complete. FFQs are analyzed by computer for saturated fat and cholesterol content. At the same time, the computer generates a personalized Nutrition Progress Report which provides feedback to the patient regarding his or her intake of saturated fat and cholesterol, suggestions for change, and food-specific goals. Other food frequency assessment tools that are appropriate and available for use in the cardiac population are listed on page 75.

Dietary Intervention

Dietary change can take months, or even years, to accomplish. Motivated individuals can make changes more quickly. Studies of post-MI patients have demonstrated high motivation among this population and good success in changing diet in a relatively short time (i.e., 3 to 12 weeks) (Kris-Etherton, et al., 1988). Therefore, health care professionals can be quite aggressive with dietary intervention during the early weeks or months after the cardiac event, using follow-up contacts to work on maintenance strategies. For example, it is perfectly appropriate to insist the post-MI patient stop eating meat at breakfast and lunch. After just a week or two, this same patient may be asked to cut the evening meat portion in half. So in just one month, a patient progresses from a steady diet of meat to the recommended limit of three ounces per day. Maintenance counseling should begin promptly by working with the patient to anticipate and plan for the situations that might cause relapse to the old pattern.

There are two distinct aspects to dietary change that the health professional should address during the intervention:

- The individual food items that the patient consumes
- The lifestyle or behavior patterns that promote consumption of these items

Lifestyle Patterns

Examples of lifestyle patterns that could be problematic include shopping at mini-marts (where low-fat foods are not available), reliance on fast-food establishments for meals, and purchasing lunch at work rather than bringing it from home. Dietary assessment tools help identify the food items that can be targeted for change, while more informal methods (conversation and interview) can be used to assess lifestyle patterns that can be modified. Typical questions for assessing lifestyle patterns are listed below.

Frequency of eating

How many meals and snacks do you usually eat?

Involvement with food

Who does the cooking and shopping in your household?

Snacking patterns

When and where do you snack?
Where does the snack come from (coworker, vending machine, bakery, etc.)?

Eating out

How often do you eat out?
Where do you go and what do you order?

Social eating

Do you often arrange to see friends over: A meal? Coffee and dessert? Drinks and appetizers?

Business eating

Does your work involve: Business lunches? Breakfast meetings? Cocktail receptions?

Formulating Goals

Health care professionals can facilitate the dietary change process by providing specific, personalized advice and information regarding food choices and patterns. Although it may be helpful for the health care professional to know exactly how much total fat, saturated fat, and cholesterol the patient consumes, this information is of secondary relevance for the patient. Patients are more likely to respond to specific food messages such as "have meat no more than two or three times per week" than to nutrient messages such as "limit fat to 40 grams per day."

With this in mind, the health care professional can evaluate an individual's diet, using either food records or food frequencies for the "big-ticket items"—foods providing the greatest proportion of saturated fat and cholesterol for that particular patient. These may include moderately fatty foods, such as chips and cookies, that are eaten on a daily basis, or very fatty foods, such as pizza and ice cream, that are eaten several times a week. Red meats are almost always among the "big-ticket items" in a typical American diet and should be targeted for change from the start.

Prioritizing Goals

The health professional should prioritize the desirable food changes for a patient based on his or her customary intake. Of top priority are the food changes that would reduce saturated fat and cholesterol intake the most; the middle set of changes would reduce them to a lesser extent; low-priority changes are those that would be beneficial but significantly less dramatic than the other changes. These recommended food changes should be presented to the patient as goals; in other words, as specific and measurable food-related behaviors to be accomplished in a given time frame.

Examples of suitable goals include:

> *"Reduce red meat portions to 3 ounces (the size of a deck of cards)."*

> *"Limit egg yolks to four per week."*

> *"Switch to fat-free salad dressing."*

In most cases, a suitable time frame for accomplishing initial goals is approximately two weeks.

The prioritized list of goals can serve as a starting point for discussions between patient and professional. Patients should be permitted to modify goals and to select several (about three) that he or she feels confident pursuing right away. Goals should always be realistic and attainable so that the patient does not become discouraged. In follow-up contacts, goal attainment can be evaluated, and new goals can be added or old ones revised until a satisfactory diet is reached. A "satisfactory diet" is one that is similar to the National Cholesterol Education Program Step 2 diet containing less than 30% of calories from fat, less than 7% from saturated fat, and less than 200 mg of cholesterol daily.

Self-Efficacy

When assessing baseline dietary patterns, it is also worthwhile to assess each patient's self-efficacy for change by asking, for example, "On a scale of 0 to 100, how confident are you that you can limit yourself to two or fewer egg yolks per week?" (See the sample "Efficacy Questionnaire" on p. 76.) A score of 80 or more would indicate high self-efficacy, suggesting that the patient could set a goal of two or fewer eggs per week with a reasonable chance of meeting the goal immediately. A score of 70 or less indicates an area where patients might be more successful making step-wise or slower changes; for example, cutting usual egg consumption in half rather than all the way down to two eggs per week. If the patient is successful after a month or so, he or she could then cut the weekly number of eggs in half again until the goal of two eggs per week is reached.

Attitudes and Feelings

From the health care professional's point of view, dietary change follows the basic steps set forth in the problem-solving model discussed in chapter 2.

From the patient's point of view, the process may be considerably more complicated. Changing dietary patterns may be perceived as painful, socially disruptive, expensive, and laborious. It may bring up images of deprivation, domestic turmoil, loss of identity, and loss of pleasure. The health care professional can begin to assess these attitudes and concerns in early conversations so that the negative feelings are addressed and dispelled as soon as possible. Dietitians, doctors, nurses, and other health care professionals who have themselves adopted low-fat eating patterns can be especially effective in helping the patient develop positive attitudes and skills for necessary dietary changes.

Building Skills

Besides addressing the behavioral and lifestyle patterns of the patient, dietary intervention must also address certain skills related to food. These skills include cooking with less fat, reading food labels, ordering low-fat meals in restaurants, and making suitable trade-offs to keep food interesting and enjoyable.

There are some excellent low-fat cookbooks that can be recommended to patients. Health care professionals can help by providing an annotated list of suitable books that are available locally. Dietitians frequently have current knowledge of such resources and may be able to compile the list with little effort. A sample "List of Cookbooks" appears on p. 77.

It would require a full-time effort to keep up with all the different food products and formulations one might encounter in the grocery store. As an alternative, health care professionals can train patients to read and interpret product labels for relevant information regarding the types and amount of fat in foods. The new food labeling requirements, effective May 1994, make the relevant information much easier to obtain.

Similar information in a similar format may be displayed at meat counters for the major cuts of meat and poultry. Patients should be encouraged to take advantage of this information and to choose the leanest cuts of meat possible. The labeling of meat and poultry is not mandatory, however, and patients may need to request the information from the store manager.

In general, patients can be directed to food products falling below the limits set forth in Table 6.1. In practice, however, it is not enough for patients to know the grams of fat, saturated fat, and cholesterol in a food product. They need to

Table 6.1   Guidelines for Acceptable Fat Content in Processed Foods

	Snack foods & side dishes	Frozen dinners & prepared meals
Total fat	< 5 g/serving	< 10 g/serving
Saturated fat	Approx. 1 g/serving	< 2.5 g/serving
Cholesterol	< 25 mg/serving	< 50 mg/serving
Sodium (1- to 2-g daily limit)	< 80 mg/serving	< 200 mg/serving

understand this information in the context of how often they eat the food, how much of it they eat each time, and what else they are eating.

Similarly, we can help patients learn to interpret restaurant menus and develop skills for finding and ordering foods that are consistent with the dietary plan. The requisite skills go beyond the culinary arena to the interpersonal, including the ability to be assertive and persuasive. Patients who travel frequently may need additional instruction for coping with in-flight meals. Others may need help learning to deal with business affairs and social eating.

Co-Morbid Conditions

Many cardiac patients have the added complication of having to balance a heart-healthy diet with other dietary requirements (e.g., diabetic, low sodium, or renal requirements). Patients will have better success with dietary management if all the diet requirements are addressed in a single plan instead of being treated separately. This will require the help of a trained dietitian.

Follow-Up and Repeat Assessments

Follow-up contacts are an important aspect of dietary management. Many unforseen questions and problems arise that must be addressed in follow-up if the patient is to succeed with his or her behavior change program. Follow-up should focus on goals and on problem solving. Dietary assessment should be incorporated into the follow-up regimen for several reasons:

- To determine what positive changes have been made so they can be reinforced by the health care professional
- To determine if negative changes have been made that require correcting (such as substituting cheese for red meat)
- To determine if new, more aggressive goals can be set

Ideally, follow-up assessments employ the same tools and evaluation method originally used to measure dietary intake. If resources are limited, however, interim assessments can focus on the dietary goals that the patient has set. For example, if the patient set goals for limiting consumption of eggs, fast foods, and ice cream, then assessment can focus on the patient's consumption of these items during the week prior to follow-up. Patient recall or weekly tally sheets can be used for these simplified assessments. Be aware that assessments that measure only goal-related foods will not accomplish the second purpose of repeat assessments, which is to identify backsliding or negative changes, and may not help with the third purpose of adding new, more aggressive goals. Health care professionals should probe for dietary change information that might not surface if only goal attainment is assessed.

Dietary follow-up can be expedited by substituting telephone contacts for face-to-face visits. Any printed feedback regarding dietary intake or goal attainment can be mailed to the patient prior to the contact. Telephone contacts are usually initiated by the health care professional at a prearranged day and time, as noted in chapter 3.

Maintenance

Maintenance of dietary change is important for the long-term management of coronary heart disease. There is a growing body of research data on dietary maintenance, although at present the data are insufficient to draw firm conclusions. Certain parallels drawn from the weight management arena indicate that dietary change is better maintained when social and lifestyle issues are addressed as part of the dietary change program (Block, 1982).

Dietary maintenance is enhanced when the changes identified and made are appropriate in the first place—that is, when they are changes that the patient can tolerate and be satisfied with permanently. This usually means reducing rather than eliminating foods, and accommodating occasional intake of favorite foods even though they may be high in fat.

Maintenance counseling can then focus on the foods and situations that are most likely to cause proper eating patterns to deteriorate. These foods and situations will vary for each individual, but should be fairly clear to the patient after 3 to 6 months of dietary intervention. At this point, the patient may be asked to list the two or three foods and the two or three situations that are likely to be problematic, and to propose strategies for addressing these specific situations. During counseling for maintenance, the health care professional should strive to ensure three things: that the patient has set realistic maintenance goals, that he or she has a plan for recognizing slips, and that he or she has a plan for correcting them.

Intervention Summary and Model

To summarize, the dietary change program includes the following:

- Assessing dietary intake
- Assessing lifestyle patterns
- Assessing self-efficacy for change
- Prioritizing dietary changes based on assessments
- Solving problems that involve lifestyle patterns
- Addressing negative feelings and attitudes about dietary change
- Working with the patient to set specific, attainable, short-term goals based on assessments
- Referring patients to a dietitian when multiple dietary restrictions apply
- Building skills (label reading, food preparation, eating out, etc.)
- Evaluating goal attainment and revising or adding goals
- Providing maintenance counseling

Each of these tasks can be accomplished by a rehabilitation specialist, assuming there are adequate tools and resources for assessing the diet. If not, a dietitian may help with this first task. Counseling and education traditionally take place face-to-face, in either individual or group situations. Both channels are generally effective, but they are not always available, affordable, or convenient for all patients and all health care facilities. Alternative models which are less reliant on face-to-face contact may be appealing to some patients and in some settings.

One such model is the Computer-Assisted Learning System (CALS), which was developed and tested by the Stanford Cardiac Rehabilitation Program. CALS incorporates the dietary intervention elements into a cohesive program that takes advantage of computer technology to accommodate large numbers of patients and to require minimal staff resources. CALS has been tested on 835 hyper-cholesterolemic patients, with an overall cholesterol reduction of 5 to 7% over a period of 3 to 6 months. Dramatic changes in dietary intake of saturated fat and cholesterol are typically noted after 4 to 6 weeks and maintained after 3 to 6 months (Clark, DeBusk, Johansson, Hyman, & Corsetto, 1988).

The CALS program consists of the following:

- Food Frequency Questionnaires to assess dietary intake of saturated fat and cholesterol at baseline, 4, and 8 weeks
- A baseline self-efficacy assessment
- Individualized computer-generated feedback reports following each FFQ
- A dietary workbook offering specific food and nutrition information, self-assessment and planning tools, and behaviorally oriented instruction

The ''CALS Dietary Intervention Components and Examples'' are listed on p. 78. We have used CALS successfully with varying levels of interaction. In MULTIFIT, nurses provided face-to-face counseling at baseline with telephone follow-up after each feedback report. In an HMO setting, a health educator provided baseline dietary counseling with CALS. In both HMO and worksite settings, CALS was administered alone. Cholesterol levels dropped a dramatic 14% in MULTIFIT as a result of multiple lifestyle interventions. Applications of CALS in isolation lowered blood cholesterol by between 5 and 7% (Clark, DeBusk, Johansson, Hyman, & Corsetto, 1988).

Weight Management

Weight management for the cardiac patient has two aspects:

- Weight loss for patients who are overweight
- Prevention of future weight gain for everyone except the underweight patient

Overweight patients should be encouraged to lose weight, and a goal of 4.5 kg (10 lb) is suitable for lowering blood pressure and blood cholesterol levels. Although many patients can afford to lose much more than 4.5 kg, it is not realistic to expect that they will. Despite the many programs and studies devoted to weight loss, the fact remains that there are few successes to report. We therefore focus on the 4.5 kg reduction in order to improve risk factors associated with heart disease. Patients who can achieve and maintain a 4.5 kg loss may want to lose more, and the health care professional should certainly encourage the effort. Patients should be cautioned to lose only as much weight as they can comfortably maintain.

The exercise training and low-fat dietary programs recommended for cardiac patients often result in modest weight loss. In fact, it has been shown that substituting low-fat foods for higher fat ones can result in a weight reduction of 2.5 kg (5.6 lb) in just 11 weeks, even when the total amount of food is not restricted (Kendall, Levitsky, Strupp, & Lissner, 1991). Health care professionals who gloss over the diet issue in patient counseling should be encouraged by this fact, for it greatly simplifies dietary instruction for the cardiac patient. The weight management approach can be as simple as regulating the fat content of the diet. Adding another simple dimension—frequency of eating—yields a fairly comprehensive weight control plan. Simply stated, the dietary guidelines for weight management are as follows:

- Eat three meals every day in order to avoid overeating and binge-eating.
- Limit snacks to 2 or 3 per day.
- Stick with low-fat foods as much as possible.
- Follow the prescribed exercise program.

Health care professionals should monitor body weight and use small successes, such as losing a few pounds in the early months of treatment, as incentives for the patient to maintain the lifestyle changes that contributed to the loss and to further accelerate his or her efforts if appropriate.

At the very least, the cardiac patient should be monitoring his or her weight in order to prevent the gradual weight gain that most Americans experience with age. Patients can be advised to take immediate action (such as increasing exercise or seeking help) whenever a weight increase of any amount persists for more than a month.

Summary

Dietary intervention should identify and address the foods and the lifestyle patterns that contribute to a high-fat, high-cholesterol diet. The health care professional may need to address food-related attitudes and beliefs, in addition to knowledge and skill levels. Goals for each patient should be specific and realistic, and goal attainment should be evaluated periodically so remedial measures can be taken if necessary.

Mia Clark is nutritionist and writer with the Stanford Cardiac Rehabilitation Program. She has developed applications for dietary assessment and feedback including an interactive version known as DietCoach™.

Sample Questions
From the Food Frequency Questionnaire

Part I. We want to know how often you ate certain foods. For each of the foods listed, please indicate how many servings per week you *usually* ate in the past month. (If you ate a food less than once a week, write a ''0'' in the space provided.) Where indicated, check whether your servings were large, small, or about average in size.

Food item	Average weekly servings	Serving size: Lg.	Av.	Sm.	Size of average serving
Red meat (beef, pork and ham, veal, lamb)	____	____	____	____	4 ounces
Meat dishes (casseroles, tacos, pizza, meat sauce)	____	____	____	____	1 cup casserole, 1 taco or pizza slice
Chicken or turkey	____	____	____	____	1 lg or 2 sm pieces
Fish or shellfish, including fish canned in water	____	____	____	____	4 ounces, 1/2 can
Bacon, sausage	____	____	____	____	2 pieces

****

Food item	Average weekly servings	Size of average serving
Whole eggs or egg yolks	____	1 egg or yolk
Milk, yogurt, or cottage cheese	____	1 cup (8 ounces)
Cheese or cream cheese	____	1 ounce/slice
Ice cream	____	1/2 cup (1 scoop)
Fruits, fresh or dried	____	1 whole piece or 1 cup cut-up fruit

****

Part II. For each of the following items, check the *one* answer that best describes you. Use your eating habits of the past month as your standard.

Between butter and margarine,

___ 1. I almost always use butter.

___ 2. I almost always use margarine.

___ 3. I use both.

___ 4. I don't use butter or margarine.

The person who cooks my food

___ 1. almost always uses butter, shortening, or lard for cooking and baking.

___ 2. almost always uses vegetable oil or margarine for cooking and baking.

___ 3. uses both butter, shortening, or lard *and* vegetable oil or margarine.

___ 4. doesn't use any fat at all for cooking and baking.

When I use milk,

___ 1. I almost always use whole milk.

___ 2. I use both whole and lowfat (2%) milk.

___ 3. I almost always use lowfat (2%) milk.

___ 4. I use both lowfat (2%) and nonfat (skim) milk, or 1% milk.

___ 5. I almost always use nonfat (skim) milk.

___ 6. I don't use milk.

When I eat chicken or turkey,

___ 1. I almost always eat the skin.

___ 2. I almost never eat the skin.

___ 3. I sometimes eat the skin.

___ 4. I don't eat chicken or turkey.

When I eat meat, fish, or poultry,

___ 1. I almost always have it fried or cooked with oil or another fat, or with gravy.

___ 2. I almost always have it broiled, baked, or stewed, and without any gravy or fat.

___ 3. I have it prepared in both fashions listed above.

___ 4. I don't eat meat, fish, or poultry.

****

Food Frequency Assessment Tools

- **The Quantitative Food Frequency Analysis** was developed by Blanken-horn, Johnson, and Selzer at the University of Southern California, and is currently available as the "Quick Check for Saturated Fat" from Nutrition Scientific, 1510 Oxley St., Suite F, South Pasadena, CA 91030. This instrument can be analyzed using an IBM-compatible computer and provides feedback to the patient on saturated fat, total fat, and cholesterol intake.
- **Harvard-Willett Food Frequency Questionnaire**, developed by W.C. Willet, MD, is a much longer and more comprehensive questionnaire that measures a broad spectrum of nutrients, including total calories, total fat, saturated fat, polyunsaturated fat, cholesterol, and sodium. The standardized form is computer-analyzed to produce a list of intake levels for the various nutrients. Further information on the tool is available from Laura Sampson at the Channing Laboratory, Harvard Medical School, Boston, MA 02115.
- **The Block Questionnaires**, developed by Block (1982), have taken various forms. There is a very short 13-item version that was originally a screening tool to detect high (or low) fat intake. The longer, more comprehensive versions are interviewer administered and sensitive to a number of nutrients. For information, contact Gladys Block at the School of Public Health, University of California at Berkeley, Berkeley, CA 94710.
- **The Diet Habit Survey** of Connor, et al. (1992) was specifically designed to identify dietary habits related to coronary heart disease and to track changes in these habits. There is a self-scoring version of the questionnaire, as well as research and clinical versions. The questionnaire yields scores for cholesterol-saturated fat, carbohydrates, beverages, restaurants/recipes, and sodium. The questionnaire is available from Heart Studies Publications, Oregon Health Sciences University - L465, 3181 S.W. Sam Jackson Park Rd., Portland, OR 97201-3098.

Efficacy Questionnaire

Please rate your confidence that you can achieve and stick to the eating habits described below during the coming month. Rate your confidence for each of the 16 items with a *number* from the following scale:

0	10	20	30	40	50	60	70	80	90	100
Definitely			Probably		Maybe		Probably			Definitely
cannot			cannot		(50/50)		can			*can*
do it										do it

CONFIDENCE   *Use a number between 0 and 100*

____ 1. I can limit the amount of meat I eat to two to three small servings per week.

____ 2. I can limit the amount of chicken I eat to five small servings per week or less.

____ 3. I can limit how often I eat bacon and sausage to once per week or less.

____ 4. I can limit how often I eat hot dogs and luncheon meat to once per week or less.

____ 5. I can limit fast foods to twice per week or less.

____ 6. I can switch to nonfat or 1% fat milk and yogurt.

____ 7. I can limit myself to two or fewer egg yolks per week.

____ 8. I can limit how often I eat cheese to twice per week or less.

____ 9. I can limit the amount of ice cream I eat to two servings per week or less.

____ 10. I can limit rich breads (biscuits, croissants, bakery muffins) to once per week or less.

____ 11. I can limit salad dressing to one serving (2 tbsp) per day.

____ 12. I can limit my use of spreads (butter, margarine, and mayonnaise) to 3 tsp per day.

____ 13. I can limit how often I eat nuts or peanut butter to three times per week or less.

____ 14. I can limit myself to one or two servings of chips and/or fries per week.

____ 15. I can limit donuts and sweet rolls to once per week or less.

____ 16. I can limit the amount of high-fat sweets (cookies, cake, candy bars, etc.) I eat to two or less per week.

List of Cookbooks and Food Magazines

Recommended Cookbooks

New American Diet, by Sonja and William Connor, published by Simon & Schuster, NY. Here is a guide to making gradual dietary changes, complete with weight loss tips, menus, and lots of recipes. Most, but not all of the recipes are quite low in fat and cholesterol.

Eater's Choice, by Ron and Nancy Goor, published by Houghton Mifflin, NY. This is an all-purpose cholesterol-lowering resource. The first 100-plus pages are devoted to relevant health and nutrition information, followed by a wide variety of recipes for all occasions. Most recipes are relatively low in fat. Recipes are labeled with total calories and saturated fat calories per serving. The book includes nutrient tables for common foods.

Don't Eat Your Heart Out, 1982; *Choices for a Healthy Heart*, 1987; and *Controlling Your Fat Tooth*, 1990; all written by Joseph C. Piscatella and published by Workman Publishing, NY. These books provide practical and reliable information on all aspects of a healthy lifestyle and have built-in behavior modification tips. The recipes are generally simple and quite low in fat and cholesterol. The books (especially the first one) can provide motivation for patients in that they recount the author's own battle with heart disease and lifestyle change.

Deliciously Low, 1983; and *Deliciously Simple*, 1986; by Harriet Roth, published by New American Library, NY. Both of these cookbooks contain recipes that are easy to prepare and low in fat and cholesterol. Recipes are well labeled with nutrient information.

Entertaining Light, 1991; *Mediterranean Light*, 1989; and *Provençal Light*, 1994; by Martha Rose Shulman, published by Bantam Books, NY. These books are suitable for gourmet and special-occasion cooking. Not every recipe is very low in fat, but each recipe is labeled with nutrient information (including total fat, cholesterol, and sodium) so the reader can make informed choices.

Recommended Magazines

A magazine subscription is a good way to periodically renew enthusiasm for new and different recipes.

Cooking Light: The Magazine of Food and Fitness. P.O. Box C-549, Birmingham, AL 35282. Or call 1-800-633-8628. The recipes are low in fat and calories. The stunning photographs make the magazine a pleasure to read.

Eating Well, The Magazine of Food & Health. Ferry Rd., P.O. Box 1001, Charlotte, VT 05445-9977. Each issue contains reliable information about foods and health, as well as low-fat recipes and cooking tips.

Computer-Assisted Learning System (CALS) Dietary Intervention Components and Examples

Intervention component	Example from CALS model
Assessing dietary intake	Food frequency questionnaire (FFQ)
Assessing lifestyle patterns	Self-assessment quizzes in workbook
Assessing self-efficacy	Confidence rating
Prioritizing dietary changes	Priorities set by computer, based on FFQ responses and confidence levels
Applying problem-solving techniques to lifestyle patterns	Workbook exercises
Addressing feelings and attitudes	Face-to-face or telephone contact
Goal-setting (short term)	Computer feedback and workbook
Referring the patient to other health care professionals as needed	Face-to-face and/or telephone follow-up
Skill-building	Workbook instruction
Evaluating and revising goals	Repeat FFQ and computer feedback
Maintaining lifestyle changes	Computerized feedback of maintenance goals based on changes that were made

Chapter 7

Stress Management

F ew issues in cardiovascular risk analysis are as controversial as the importance of stress. The controversy arises in part because of the difficulty of measuring stress. While researchers may argue about the importance of stress, surveys show that the public feels that it is one of the most important causes of heart disease. In a survey of the patients participating in our home exercise training trial (DeBusk et al., 1985), we found that about half believed their heart attack was caused by stress. The public's interest in stress, alone, is sufficient justification for its inclusion in a lifestyle modification program. One survey of 173 cardiac rehabilitation programs found that only 25% offered stress management (Thomas et al., in press). But what should be the focus of a stress management program, and how should stress management be taught?

Stress and Cardiovascular Disease

Many years ago, Friedman and Rosenman (1959) suggested that Type A behavior is associated with an increased risk of death from coronary heart disease. In subsequent studies (Rosenman et al., 1975), they found that men who exhibited the TABP (Type A Behavior Pattern)—characterized by extreme competitiveness; excessive drive; free-floating hostility; enhanced sense of time-urgency; multitasking; and rapid, interruptive speech—were much more likely to die from CHD than men without these features. A 1978 consensus conference of researchers in the field concluded that there was sufficient evidence to support the role of TABP as an independent risk factor for CHD, and the risk was as great as other conventional risk factors (The Review Panel on Coronary-Prone Behavior and Coronary Heart Disease, 1981). However, many subsequent studies have found either no, or weak, relationships with global TABP and other CHD risk factors, morbidity, or mortality (Shuster et al., 1992).

In recent years, studies have begun to focus on the components of Type A behavior most strongly related to CHD. Of these, the factor most closely related to CHD seems to be some aspect of anger/hostility. Hostility, measured by scales such as the Cook-Medley scale, has been strongly correlated with morbidity and mortality from CHD (Barefoot, Dahlstrom, & Williams, 1983; Williams, Haney, Lee, Kong, Blumenthal, & Whalen, 1980). Reexamination of data from both the Western Collaborative Group Study and the MRFIT trial revealed evidence of a markedly elevated risk of CHD in the hostile patient groups (Dembroski,

MacDougall, Costa, & Grandits, 1989; Hecker, Chesney, Black, & Frautschi, 1988). This is especially impressive since the MRFIT data showed no evidence of increased CHD risk associated with global ratings of TABP. Anger/hostility may have both a long-term and immediate effect on CHD function. Anger is a potent psychological stressor in patients with CHD, leading to adverse changes in physiology such as decreased ejection fraction in at-risk individuals (Ironson et al., 1992). Yet the nature of the anger/hostility remains vague. It is not clear if the important function is suppressed anger/hostility, cynicism, potential for hostility, acute anger, and/or repeated anger.

Perhaps the most impressive data on the importance of TABP or some component of TABP comes from studies that have attempted to modify it. Friedman et al. (1986) randomly assigned 862 patients to group cardiac counseling focusing on behavior modification of Type A, or to a control group that received regular cardiac counseling only. TABP was significantly reduced in the treatment group. At follow-up 4.5 years later, the TABP treatment group had 12.9% nonfatal MIs and cardiac deaths compared to 21.2% in the control group (Friedman et al., 1986). Ornish et al. (1990) also evaluated the impact of stress management and other risk factor modifications on CHD. Twenty-eight patients with CHD received 24 days of training in stress management (stretching and relaxation, meditation, visualization, and environmental manipulation), smoking cessation, an exercise program, and a modified vegetarian diet. A control group received routine care. The intervention led to slight regression of coronary atherogenesis as measured by angiography, while progression occurred in the control group. Since the intervention was multifactorial, it is not possible to determine the specific effects of stress management. However, these two studies provide evidence of possible impact of intensive stress management on the reduction of CHD morbidity. A third study has also demonstrated the effects of stress management on CHD in post-MI patients, and provides a more workable model. Frasure-Smith and Prince (1989) randomly assigned patients to supportive treatment after MI, or to no treatment. In this simple treatment program, nurses used the General Health Questionnaire to assess patients' level of stress and emotional discomfort during telephone calls. Patients who exhibited stress were then visited at home for stress management and support directed at reducing stress. At 1 year after treatment, there was a reduction in cardiac death rates of about 50%.

Stress caused by upsetting life events and sustained demands that tax or exceed a person's ability and resources to cope is also important in risk-factor modification. Stressors are an important component of relapse. For instance, many ex-smokers report relapsing during stressful situations. Many individuals eat excessively while under stress, fail to adhere to programs when overwhelmed by stress, and simply feel bad while under stress. This type of stress is usually defined in terms of psychological demands exceeding a person's coping resources; stress related to CHD, on the other hand, takes a more chronic form, that is, the Type A Behavior Pattern or some component of it. Essentially the same stress management techniques are used for both problems, however.

A Model for Stress Management

There is vast literature reporting the results of various types of stress management interventions for improving a variety of physiological and psychological problems, such as headaches. This literature indicates that fairly simple interventions that include some type of relaxation procedure likely to induce the so-called relaxation response (Benson, 1976) produce the most cost-effective benefits. We recommend a model in which education about stress is combined with simple techniques appropriate for everyone. Individuals failing to respond are referred to more intensive stress reduction programs. The assumptions behind our model are as follows:

- Patients with cardiovascular disease need and want to learn about stress, stress management, and anger/hostility.
- Simple, common-sense information and instructions about managing stress in one's life has a positive impact for most individuals.
- Relaxation tapes are a useful tool for stress management.
- Some individuals need more intensive stress management than can be obtained from the more simple, cost-effective techniques.
- Patients should be instructed on how to monitor stress in their lives, and should be encouraged to seek more intensive help if necessary.
- Stress management must be tailored to the individual's problems and issues, and to situations involving a high risk of relapse, nonadherence, nonparticipation, etc.
- Stress management must be practiced regularly.

The Stress Management Intervention

In our first multifactorial intervention, we developed an intensive six-session audiovisual stress management program accompanied by a short manual called "Staying Cool." This program was very popular with our patients and became the basis for the stress management component of MULTIFIT and the Active Partnership™ program. The components of the MULTIFIT intervention are as follows:

a. Baseline evaluation of perceived stress and patient's desire for help in this area

b. Active Partnership™ stress management video

c. Stress management section of the Active Partnership™ workbook

d. Active Partnership™ relaxation tape

e. Monitoring of stress during telephone calls

f. Referral for more intensive intervention as needed

Baseline Evaluation

The MULTIFIT intervention begins with a simple baseline evaluation of the patient's perceived level of stress using the questions embedded in the Psychosocial Questionnaire (see p. 38). This information, usually obtained 2 to 3 days after admission, is used to identify patients who may have intense levels of anxiety, stress, or tension. Because patients often experience stress as tension and anxiety, we ask if patients are feeling either anxious or panicky. On follow-up calls, special attention is paid to individuals who report moderate or higher levels of tension, anxiety, stress, or pressure at baseline to ensure that they are receiving the help needed or that they are referred for further help as needed.

There are more elaborate ways to measure stress and the impact of stress on an individual. A number of instruments have been developed to assess both stress and coping. These include the Cohen Stress Scale (Cohen, Kamarck, & Mermelstein, 1983) and the Coping Responses Inventory (Moos, 1988), which can be easily administered in rehabilitation settings.

Active Partnership™ Stress Management Video

All patients are shown the Active Partnership™ stress management video while in hospital. The main purpose of the video is to help patients understand what stress is, how it affects them, and how it can be managed. The videotape follows three patients through their days, observing the stressors they encounter. Viewers are then shown how these patients might alter, adapt, or avoid those stressors.

Active Partnership™ Workbook

Following the film, all patients are instructed to review the stress management section of the Active Partnership™ workbook. Our goal in the workbook is to present the most important general concepts about stress. We believe that many patients can make major improvements in how they cope with stress through relatively simple changes in their lives, beginning with a commitment to lead a less stressful life. Much of the change is based on common sense and the belief that, given the opportunity, most people can readily identify the areas most stressful to them and can use their own experience in improving the situation.

As part of the workbook, subjects use a checklist to help them identify problems they may be having with stress. Individuals are also encouraged to keep track of their stress by keeping a stress diary for at least a week. The goal of the diary is to make patients more aware of stressors in their lives and their responses to them. Following a week of keeping the stress diary, patients are given four basic ways of coping with stress:

1. Learning to relax by following the relaxation audiotape
2. Using emergency stress stoppers such as counting to 10 before speaking when angry
3. Exercising
4. Reducing chemical stressors such as smoking and caffeine

Patients are then instructed (a) to learn to avoid stressors as needed and appropriate; (b) to learn to alter stressors, beginning with an appraisal of what a person can realistically do to change the stressor; (c) to learn to adapt to situations by changes in attitude, response, or behavior; (d) to learn some basic assertiveness or speaking-up skills; and (e) to practice better time management. These five skills encompass most of what is practiced in more intensive face-to-face group programs, many individual therapy programs, and self-help materials.

The manual concludes with a very brief section on problem solving. Patients often need more help with problem solving than is available using written material alone. Thus the focus of the telephone calls conducted by the nurses is on individual problem solving.

There are many other self-help stress management materials available, and no studies have been conducted demonstrating the superiority of one over another. The health care professional should choose written materials that fit his or her philosophy, that would seem to be effective if no outcome data is available on them, and that are easily used and understood by patients.

Active Partnership™ Relaxation Audiotape

The Active Partnership™ relaxation audiotape uses standard relaxation instructions. Benson, Beary, and Carol (1974), building on work by Gellhorn (1970), observed that progressive muscle relaxation, hypnosis, and many forms of meditation shared several properties: the subject assumes a passive frame of mind in a relaxing position, repeats a simple phrase, and breathes in a deep, regular manner. They argued that this elicits the "relaxation response," which tends to reduce central nervous system sympathetic activity. Since the relaxation response can be induced in rather simple ways, cost, convenience, and patient preference should be strong considerations in how to make this a component of a program. We favor the use of a relaxation tape, which we encourage patients to listen to every day for the first month, and then as needed thereafter. Some patients prefer biofeedback; others like hypnosis or meditation. All of these techniques seem to achieve the same benefit.

Using Telephone Calls to Monitor Stress

After the patients have seen the videotape, asked questions, and begun using the audiotape and workbook, we use telephone calls to monitor how they are doing. At each call, the nurses are instructed to ask the following questions:

1. *How have you been feeling emotionally since we last talked?*

   No problems   _____

   Depressed   _____

   Anxious   _____

   Stressed   _____

2. *Has anything happened to you that has been very upsetting?*

No   _____

Yes   _____

Based on the patient's response, the nurse answers the following question and follows through as needed:

3. *Does the patient need a referral for counseling?*

No   _____

Yes   _____ (Complete a referral and log it onto the physician referral log.)

The telephone call is an integral part of stress management, allowing us to monitor how patients are doing and to provide assistance or referral as needed.

Referral

Most patients who follow this program improve their coping skills. However, a few patients require more intensive intervention because they continue to have incapacitating symptoms or distress. Such people may benefit from more intensive interventions provided by specialists. Rehabilitation personnel should identify health professionals in the community who can provide such interventions. Most patients readily accept referral.

Measuring Outcomes

Measuring the effectiveness of stress management programs is difficult and no standard instrument exists. Coordinators of cardiac rehabilitation programs may need to design their own evaluation tools to assess patient satisfaction with the stress management program, perceived benefit of the program, and other items.

Summary

Although the significance of stress as a risk factor in CHD remains controversial, many patients view stress management as an important part of their recovery. Moreover, stress caused by upsetting events and extra demands decreases a patient's ability to effectively modify their lifestyle. To ensure adequate rehabilitation, it is critical to assess patients' stress using standard or clinical instruments, to offer simple interventions such as relaxation techniques, to monitor patients' stress levels, and to refer patients to more intensive programs when necessary.

Chapter 8

Smoking Cessation

S moking is the single most important cause of preventable death in the United States today. When treating the patient with cardiovascular disease who smoked prior to hospitalization, increased attention must be given to this risk factor during hospitalization in order to provide the patient with skills necessary to maintain cessation. This chapter highlights a stepped approach to helping patients quit smoking. This approach is behaviorally oriented and offers additional information about the importance of nicotine replacement therapy.

Risks and Benefits

Continued smoking after a coronary event is associated with an increased rate of morbidity and mortality. For example, patients who continue to smoke after an MI experience twice the mortality of those who stop (Wilhelmsson, Vedin, Elmfeldt, Tibblin, & Wilhelmsen, 1975). Moreover, continued smoking after coronary angioplasty has been reported to be associated with an increased re-stenosis rate (Galan, Deligonul, Kern, Chaitman, & Vandormael, 1988). Smoking has also been shown to cause silent ischemia (Barry et al., 1989), to block the increase in coronary blood flow normally associated with exercise (Winniford et al., 1987), to trigger coronary spasm and abnormal segmental narrowing of the coronary arteries (Maouad et al., 1986), and to reduce the anti-ischemic effects of both calcium and beta channel blocking agents (Deanfield, Wright, Krikler, Ribeiro, & Fox, 1984).

Cessation of smoking following a coronary event such as a myocardial infarction or coronary revascularization is also associated with significant benefits for patients. For example, cessation of smoking has been shown to reduce the rates of reinfarction and death within 1 year of quitting (Sparrow & Dawber, 1978). Stopping smoking is further associated with a delay in the onset of angina (Daly, Graham, Hickey, & Mulcahy, 1985), and with an increase in HDL levels (Stubbe, Eskilsson, & Nilsson-Ehle, 1982). Finally, as noted in the Coronary Artery Surgery Study Trial (Hermanson, Omenn, Krommel, & Gersh, 1988), the reduction in risk associated with quitting smoking applies to all patients, even those above 70 years of age.

Although smoking is associated with significant increases in both morbidity and mortality in the coronary population, approximately one-third to one-half of all patients suffering a myocardial infarction will relapse to smoking within 6 to

12 months following such an event (Burling, Singleton, Bigelow, Baile, & Gottlieb, 1984). Because the overall risk of death and myocardial infarction is greater in patients with ischemic heart disease, intensive smoking intervention should be provided to these patients. In reviewing the literature, however, it appears that few randomized trials of smoking have been conducted in this population. Most of the interventions designed to help coronary patients quit smoking have included physician advice, education, or group counseling. Reported studies are generally limited by small sample size, lack uniformity regarding the definition of abstinence, and rely upon self-report data for confirmation of nonsmoking status (Burling et al., 1984). Furthermore, the proportion of "ex-smokers" defined at one point in time ("point prevalence") overestimates the sustained smoking cessation rate because detailed information regarding smoking status over an entire follow-up period has generally been unavailable.

Despite the general lack of research on intervention in the coronary population, some studies suggest that physicians and other health care professionals can have a very positive impact on smoking cessation efforts. For example, Burt et al. (1974) documented a quit rate of 63% over 3 years in patients who received firm, unequivocal advice by a physician and follow-up by nurses at the time of the MI, compared with a 27% quit rate when conventional advice was provided by a physician. In a similar randomized, controlled trial of post-MI patients, we also obtained a 71% quit rate at one year for those patients who received a nurse-managed behavioral intervention at the time of hospitalization, compared to a 45% cessation rate in those receiving usual care (Taylor, Houston Miller, Killen, & DeBusk, 1990).

Smoking Interventions

Although, after a coronary event, many smokers can quit on their own with minimal encouragement, others require some kind of formal intervention. Because combining intervention strategies appears to increase the patient's success in remaining a nonsmoker, it is our belief that multiple strategies should be employed in helping this population. Moreover, because the greatest time of relapse to smoking occurs immediately upon hospital discharge following a CHD event, intervention strategies must begin in the hospital in order to help patients prepare for potential relapse. The hospital also provides an ideal setting for a structured, individualized approach to smoking cessation because patients experience the worst part of withdrawal during the initial 48 to 72 hours after hospitalization, when smoking is forbidden.

If patients are not hospitalized for a coronary event where cessation is enforced, they may need to receive help in quitting tobacco products. Several techniques have been developed to help patients with cessation. Some programs encourage patients to reduce the number of cigarettes smoked each day by about 10% by monitoring cigarettes and cutting out the cigarettes they feel they can give up first, then progressing to actually quitting smoking. Other programs ask patients to reduce the amount of nicotine they receive by switching to brands lower in nicotine and tar before quitting. Finally, some programs ask patients to gradually reduce the amount of each cigarette smoked per day. None of these approaches appears to be more successful than the other. We like the "cold turkey" approach because it forces the patient to make a major decision, without delay, to never smoke again. Although any of these approaches can be used, it is also important to note whether or not a patient may need pharmacological therapy to help maintain cessation. Nicotine replacement therapy will be discussed in the next section.

A Stepped Approach to Smoking Cessation

We have always used a stepped approach to help patients quit smoking. Such an approach helps ensure that an adequate amount of attention has been devoted to helping patients with this particular lifestyle change. We follow these eight practical steps (Taylor & Houston Miller, 1989):

1. Provide a firm, unequivocal message.
2. Determine if the patient is willing to quit.
3. Determine the best quitting method.
4. Plan for problems associated with withdrawal.
5. Set a quit date.
6. Help the patient cope with urges to smoke.
7. Provide additional help as needed.
8. Follow up by telephone or visitation.

Provide a Firm, Unequivocal Message

Health care professionals, especially physicians, can have a very strong influence over patients by conveying a very caring, sympathetic, but firm message that the patient must stop smoking. Because smokers tend to deny or minimize anything but the clearest message, we believe this must be a very strong statement. Most physicians believe they should discuss this subject with their patients; yet they are often reluctant to do so because they do not want to alienate patients, or because they do not feel equipped to deliver the appropriate message. We have developed a script to help with such problems. This script highlights four simple statements we feel should be conveyed to the patient and gives an example of how to deliver the message. (See the "Physician Advice Statement for Smoking Cessation" on p. 95.)

Because many patients with cardiovascular disease are hospitalized and therefore are not allowed to smoke, health care professionals can address them by saying, "Because you haven't smoked in the hospital, you can now be considered a nonsmoker. As a health care professional, I must tell you that continuing to smoke most certainly will lead to further cardiovascular disease and potential death. Let's figure out how you can remain a nonsmoker."

Determine if the Patient Is Willing to Quit

As noted in the previous step, it is important to indicate to the patient why they must quit smoking. We attempt to personalize this message by associating the risks of continuing to smoke with the disease process. For example, if the patient is hospitalized for a coronary angioplasty, it is important for them to know that continued smoking has been associated with an increased restenosis rate. At this point, one can also focus on the benefits the patient may see in quitting. After providing this advice, it is important to determine if the patient is willing to try to quit smoking at this time. To measure the patient's willingness to quit smoking, we use the intention question shown below and a Likert scale for responses.

Do you intend to stay off cigarettes, or other tobacco products, in the next month?

1	2	3	4	5	6	7
Definitely no	Probably no	Possibly no	Maybe	Possibly yes	Probably yes	Definitely yes

Patients who score 3 or less are normally not interested in quitting or are not ready to quit (Taylor et al., 1988). If patients state they are not willing to quit, or if their response to a scaled question such as the one above shows that their willingness is questionable, it is important to explore their reasons for not wanting to quit and to provide solutions to any anticipated problems. If after further questioning they still have no interest in quitting, it is important to ask them to reduce the number of cigarettes or other tobacco products smoked and to ask if they are willing to be asked to try to quit in the future.

Determine the Best Quitting Method

Although it is difficult to distinguish patients who can successfully quit on their own from those who will need extra help, a person's confidence in his or her ability to quit is often a good predictor. Patients can be asked to rate their confidence in their ability to quit on their own; this can be done using a self-efficacy scale where 0 indicates no confidence and 100 equals total confidence. In our studies, patients who score less than 70 normally will have some difficulty quitting and should be offered additional support. A list of community smoking cessation programs should be made available to the patient; the list should describe the intervention methods and the cost of the program and should indicate a contact person. Patients should be asked to commit to such an intervention if services will not be provided by the rehabilitation program, hospital, or physician. Self-help materials can also be provided to patients at this time. In the MULTIFIT Program, we use the Active Partnership™ videotape, audiotape, and workbook as part of our intervention. Patients and family members are asked to view the videotape and to begin to use the workbook before hospital discharge. Occasionally, a patient may prefer to use acupuncture, hypnosis, or group programs instead of the program we offer. If the patient prefers such a program, we are pleased to help with referral and ask if we can contact the patient in a few months to see how they have done.

Plan for Problems Associated With Withdrawal

Although many patients can succeed in quitting by being involved in a group program or by participating in a behavioral intervention, some patients are highly addicted to nicotine and may need pharmacological therapy. The Fagerström Tolerance Test of Nicotine Dependence (Fagerström, 1978), an 8-item questionnaire shown on p. 96, is the most commonly used tool to measure smoking addiction. We note in our studies that patients who smoke more than 25 cigarettes per day, who smoke as soon as they get up in the morning, and who smoke when they are so ill they are in bed are highly addicted to nicotine (Tonnesen et al., 1988). Patients who have also experienced particularly troublesome withdrawal effects from cigarettes during previous attempts to quit or during a present hospitalization may also benefit from pharmacological therapy. We reserve the use of pharmacological agents for those groups of patients, or for those who relapse and who we feel could benefit from such therapy.

Pharmacological Therapy

For patients highly addicted to nicotine, pharmacological therapy in combination with behavioral strategies may enhance success with cessation. Over the years, various medications have been used to help patients counteract urges to smoke and the effects of withdrawal. At present, nicotine replacement therapy (i.e., nicotine gum or the nicotine patch) offers the greatest success rate. The use of these agents is described below.

Nicotine gum. Although the presence of cardiovascular disease is a relative contraindication to nicotine gum and the patch, physicians and patients must weigh the advantages of the patient's stopping smoking against the risks of using a medication that releases nicotine into the blood. It should be noted that blood levels obtained during the use of 2-mg nicotine gum average 12 mg/ml compared to peak levels of 35 to 50 mg/ml during smoking (Benowitz, 1988). In addition, nicotine is not released in the lungs, thereby reducing possible lung disease. We believe that the benefits of nicotine gum outweigh the risks (especially for patients without complications) for those patients who will surely smoke if not given a trial of nicotine gum. However, each CHD patient and physician must make their own decision about the risks and benefits of using nicotine gum.

One of the problems associated with nicotine gum in the past has been ineffective education about proper administration. Proper instruction, such as that given on the "Nicotine Chewing Gum Patient Information" sheet shown on p. 97, should include a prescribed, regular schedule for taking the gum so that blood nicotine levels remain constant; precautions concerning the use of acidic agents, which decrease nicotine absorption; and appropriate information about how to chew the gum and how to taper use. We find that if patients are given this type of information, their success in taking nicotine gum is enhanced and side effects are decreased.

Nicotine patch. Another pharmacological aid with promising effects is the nicotine patch. Available in the United States since December 1991, the nicotine patch is designed to be worn for a period of 16 to 24 hours, depending upon the type of patch. The patch is normally well tolerated, with minimal side effects except for local skin irritation (see the "Nicotine Transderm Patch Patient Information" sheet shown on p. 99). Unlike the gum, which, if chewed inappropriately, is not absorbed properly, the patch ensures a steady release of nicotine, which is absorbed through the skin. In most cases, the patch is designed to be worn for a period of up to 3 or 4 months, and a suggested tapering schedule is provided in the instructions. The long-term success of the nicotine patch is not yet known; however, it appears that the short-term success rates are similar to those of nicotine gum. Cessation rates range from 12 to 26% at the end of 6 months to 1 year (Hurt, Lauger, Offord, Kottke, & Dale, 1990; Transdermal Nicotine Study Group, 1991). Because the patch produces a higher serum nicotine level than the gum, its use may pose more risks for patients with coronary heart disease.

Set a Quitting Date

In order to formalize a commitment to quit smoking, we have patients sign a contract. The Active Partnership™ workbook contains a contract which formalizes an agreement, between the patient and the health care professional, to work together. As noted in chapter 2, contracts are one of the key elements in helping patients make behavior changes and can be especially useful when patients begin to undertake changes.

At this point, if a patient is to be referred to another site in the community for a specific smoking cessation program and follow-up, the physician or health care professional should consider requesting that the patient sign a contract to formalize his or her commitment to follow through. If an individualized approach using behavioral strategies is appropriate and time permits, many patients can be further counseled by health care professionals to undertake the next 3 steps.

Help the Patient Prepare to Cope With Urges to Smoke

Once a patient is formally committed to remaining an ex-smoker, preventing relapse becomes the goal of smoking cessation efforts. Because relapse is most often associated with the urge to smoke, it can be very helpful to measure the patient's confidence in the ability to resist urges to start smoking. We use the 14-item "Self-Efficacy Questionnaire on Smoking" shown on p. 100, which is a shorter version of the scale developed by Condiotte and Lichtenstein (1981). Studies have shown that self-efficacy ratings of smoking are predictive of subsequent outcome, and in the cases where smoking is resumed, specific situations are frequently predictive of the actual relapse episode (Condiotte & Lichtenstein, 1981). In our studies, a score of less than 70% confidence for a given efficacy item denotes a high risk situation (Taylor et al., 1988).

Following assessment of high risk situations, relapse prevention training involves helping patients to mobilize their resources for coping with these situations. This is accomplished by developing cognitive and behavioral strategies for a given high-risk situation and practicing coping responses through rehearsal. For instance, a patient may report only 30% confidence in his or her ability to resist the urge to smoke after a meal. Through relapse prevention training, this patient can develop techniques to handle this particular situation, such as moving away from the table after a meal, taking a walk, brushing their teeth, or focusing on the fear of chest pain as they think about their previous hospitalization. The patient is encouraged to practice these techniques even though an urge may not occur.

In the MULTIFIT program, we use the 14-item questionnaire in counseling to focus first on those efficacy items where confidence is lowest (i.e., less than 30%). Once patients feel comfortable, we move to those items between 50 and 70%. If patients achieve confidence scores greater than 70%, it is likely that they will be able to resist the temptation to smoke. Allowing patients to determine their own cognitive and behavioral strategies for managing high risk situations assures more ownership and helps the patient develop a sense of confidence in managing these situations.

Provide Additional Help as Needed

People attempting to give up smoking have a variety of concerns. For example, some patients have numerous daily stressors in their lives or encounter crises which may increase the likelihood of relapse. Others feel such a sense of loss that it almost overwhelms them. It is important to prioritize the patient's concerns and to provide individualized counseling to patients to help them better cope with giving up smoking. We define the areas needing special attention here.

Exercise

A lifestyle modification such as exercise can enhance self-control. This essentially involves replacing "negative" addictions with "positive" ones. For example, in our post-MI studies, smokers participating in an exercise training program combined with a program for cessation of smoking had greater cessation rates and smoked significantly fewer cigarettes than did those smokers not participating in the combined program (Taylor et al., 1988). In addition to the psychological benefits, regular exercise may help reduce post-cessation weight gain and minimize some withdrawal symptoms. For these reasons, we encourage patients to walk at least 10 to 15 minutes twice daily as they begin smoking cessation efforts.

Stress

Patients often relapse to smoking during extreme periods of stress or distress. Although some patients may need psychological counseling to help them cope with major life problems, relaxation training can provide many patients with a global perception of increased control, which in turn may enhance self-efficacy. For this reason, we have incorporated into our program the use of a relaxation audiotape that provides simple instructions on how to use deep breathing and muscle-tension release to achieve relaxation. Relaxation audiotapes are inexpensive and may achieve the same benefit for many patients as more elaborate or expensive procedures.

Feeling of Loss

Many patients think of giving up smoking as "losing a best friend." It is important for health care professionals who are counseling such patients to understand the magnitude of the loss associated with giving up smoking. They should acknowledge this loss and provide assistance to help patients program new activities in their lives to replace cigarette smoking. We encourage patients to focus on hobbies (old or new), and to reward themselves daily for small successes by incorporating into their daily routine positive things they enjoy.

Alcohol Abuse

Alcohol use or abuse is often a trigger for relapse. It is therefore important to determine the patient's history of alcohol use. When we make a diagnosis of alcohol abuse, we encourage the patient to seek help and recommend that alcohol abuse treatment occur simultaneously with a program for smoking cessation. We encourage heavy social drinkers to avoid alcohol or to decrease their intake substantially until they feel successful in remaining nonsmokers.

Social Support

Family and spousal support can be critical when a patient attempts to quit smoking. If family members are smokers, we encourage them to quit at the same time as the patient. In many cases, however, this is not possible, as the stress involved in other family members quitting is overwhelming. It is important, however, to initiate a plan to help the patient resist the temptation to smoke when he or she is around others, especially household members, who are doing so. We suggest that the patient ask other household members to do at least three things: (1) to refrain from smoking in their presence and, if at all possible, to smoke only outside the home; (2) to refrain from leaving cigarettes or other tobacco products lying around the house; and (3) to refrain from offering cigarettes to the patient. Family members should also be encouraged to be supportive of the patient when he or she reaches small goals on the way to quitting smoking. For example, family members should be encouraged to give the patient daily positive reinforcement for successfully quitting.

Weight Gain

Many patients are concerned about gaining weight if they quit smoking. It is now known that smokers, on average, weigh 2.25 to 4.5 kg (5 to 10 lb) less than nonsmokers. Moreover, the average weight gain upon cessation of smoking is 2.7 to 4.5 kg (6 to 10 lb), some of which is due to metabolic changes (Wack & Rodin, 1982). It appears that weight gain occurs more in those who smoke more cigarettes, have a history of weight problems, or are "restrained" eaters (Grunberg, 1982; Hall, Ginsberg, & Jones, 1986). Patients should be made aware that they are likely to gain weight upon quitting smoking, but they should be reminded that the health risks of continuing to smoke far outweigh the addition of a few pounds.

Provide Follow-Up

Patients who are attempting to quit smoking or have quit should be given support and encouragement, especially in the first 2 weeks of cessation, when the probability of relapse is highest. A call from a physician or another health care professional can make a significant difference in helping a patient. We use a structured telephone algorithm focusing on how well patients are managing cessation (see the "Telephone Interview for Patients Attempting to Quit Smoking," shown on p. 101). This telephone call is used to provide advice on how to cope with urges to smoke, to reinforce patients for their successes, and to help patients solve any additional problems they may have with their program. Follow-up telephone calls show patients that we care about them and give us feedback about the success of our program.

It is also important to determine one's success in helping patients to quit smoking. Biochemical measures such as serum and saliva thiocyanate or cotinine levels, as well as carbon monoxide (CO) readings, can be used to verify the effects of a program and to increase reliability of self-report (Cummings & Richard, 1988). Of these, serum or plasma cotinine are the most sensitive and specific. According to our standards, levels of CO > 10 ppm and/or thiocyanate > 100 mg or cotinine > 10 mg/dL indicate that a patient may be smoking. Measurement should be taken at least 6 months after cessation of smoking, once a program is completed, to ensure an adequate follow-up period.

Smoking Cessation in the MULTIFIT Program

The hospital is used as the main entryway for smoking cessation intervention in the MULTIFIT Program. Patients who have smoked in the 6 months prior to their CHD event are provided with counseling. Nurses begin by undertaking the patient's history of smoking and completing a 14-item self-efficacy scale at the bedside. Patients and family members are then shown the 16-minute Active Partnership™ videotape. This is followed by a 30-minute counseling session undertaken by the MULTIFIT nurse, primarily focused on relapse prevention training. Nurses address the issues of high-risk situations, weight gain, alcohol use, withdrawal symptoms, social support, loss and deprivation, and what to do in the event of a slip. Patients are asked to sign a contract with the nurse or a family member, formalizing their commitment to quit. Pharmacological therapy is reserved for those patients exhibiting extreme withdrawal symptoms during hospitalization. Physicians are requested to deliver a strong message, to all patients, about quitting smoking prior to discharge. All patients leave the hospital with an Active Partnership™ workbook and audiotape for use at home.

Forty-eight hours after discharge from the hospital, patients are telephoned by the nurse to inquire about their smoking status. Phone calls occur again at 14 days and 21 days, and then monthly up to 6 months. Patients who relapse into smoking at any time in this phase are offered one additional face-to-face, 30-minute counseling session if they are willing to attempt to quit again. Pharmacological therapy is initiated at this time, assuming the physician's consent is given. Additional face-to-face visits have not proven to increase success in helping patients and are not cost-effective.

Summary

A systematic approach to smoking cessation in the coronary population will lead to enhanced outcomes. Multicomponent strategies combining physician advice, educational aids, behavioral counseling, and telephone follow-up, as well as pharmacological therapy, are useful techniques which can be employed to help patients following a coronary heart disease event.

Physician Advice Statement
for Smoking Cessation

Study after study has shown that physicians play an important role in helping patients to stop smoking. Taking a few minutes to address the following four points at bedside can have a powerful influence in helping your patients to quit.

- Acknowledge that the patient smoked before hospitalization.
- Provide reinforcement for cessation of smoking during hospitalization, and indicate to the patient that he or she will have passed through the worst part of withdrawal during hospitalization, that is, in the first 2 to 3 days.
- Explain why it is important for the patient to quit smoking permanently, and personalize this message.
- Ask the patient if there is anything you can do to help him or her to remain a nonsmoker.

Here is an example of how this advice is often provided:

Mr. Jones, I know you were smoking almost a pack of cigarettes a day when you were admitted to the hospital three days ago.

I also know that it has probably been very difficult for you not to smoke since you've been here. I hope you'll take this opportunity to consider yourself an ex-smoker. You should realize that the worst period of withdrawal is during the first 2 to 3 days after quitting, and that most patients go through this period during their hospitalization.

It is important for you to quit smoking because smoking is a major risk factor that caused your coronary heart disease. Your risk is further increased because your blood pressure is high. Continuing to smoke will definitely lead to future heart problems for you.

Is there anything I can do to help you remain a nonsmoker?

Fagerström Tolerance Test of Nicotine Dependence

Questions	Answers	Points score
1. How soon after you wake do you smoke your first cigarette?	Within 30 minutes After 30 minutes	___ 1 ___ 0
2. Do you find it difficult to refrain from smoking in places where it is forbidden?	Yes No	___ 1 ___ 0
3. Which cigarette would you hate to give up the most?	The first one in the morning? Any other	___ 1 ___ 0
4. How many cigarettes do you smoke per day?	15 or less 16 to 25 26 or more	___ 0 ___ 1 ___ 2
5. Do you smoke more frequently during the early morning than during the rest of the day?	Yes No	___ 1 ___ 0
6. Do you smoke if you are so ill that you are in bed most of the day?	Yes No	___ 1 ___ 0
7. What is the nicotine level of your usual brand of cigarettes?	0.9 mg or less 1.0 to 1.2 mg 1.3 mg or more	___ 0 ___ 1 ___ 2
8. Do you inhale?	Never Sometimes Always	___ 0 ___ 1 ___ 2
	Total	___

Scoring   Scores of 7 or higher indicate high dependence on nicotine.
Scores of 6 or less indicate low to moderate nicotine dependence.

Nicotine Chewing Gum
Patient Information

PRECAUTIONS: Like all prescription drugs, THIS GUM SHOULD BE USED ONLY BY THE PERSON FOR WHOM IT HAS BEEN PRESCRIBED and SHOULD BE KEPT OUT OF THE REACH OF CHILDREN.

WARNING TO FEMALE PARTICIPANTS: DO NOT CHEW THIS GUM IF YOU ARE PREGNANT OR NURSING. This gum contains nicotine, which may cause fetal harm when chewed by a pregnant woman.Take precautions to avoid pregnancy while you are chewing this gum. If you suspect that you are pregnant, stop chewing this gum and inform us at once.

HOW THE GUM WORKS: As you chew the gum, nicotine is released and absorbed into your bloodstream through the lining in your mouth. The nicotine in the gum helps to satisfy the physical craving for nicotine and reduces nicotine withdrawal. It also replaces the oral activity of smoking, reducing the desire to smoke.

CHEWING INSTRUCTIONS:

- Chew the gum very slowly until you taste it or feel a slight tingling in your mouth. This is usually after about 15 chews, although the number is not the same for all people. The gum does not taste the same as ordinary gum.
- As soon as you get the taste of the gum, stop chewing, holding the gum in your mouth, between your cheek and gum, so the nicotine is absorbed through your cheek.
- After the taste or tingling is almost gone, after about 1 minute, chew slowly again until you taste the gum. Then stop chewing again.
- The gum should be chewed this way (off and on) for about 20 to 30 minutes to release most of the nicotine.
- Discard the gum after you have finished chewing.

During the first few weeks, we suggest you use at least one piece of gum every hour for your 12 to 16 waking hours, rather than when the smoking urge arises. DO NOT USE MORE THAN 20 PIECES OF GUM IN ONE DAY. It is very important that you not drink any liquids, especially coffee, orange juice, cola, or alcohol, just before chewing the gum (i.e., within 15 minutes of using the gum) or during the first 15 minutes of chewing the gum. These liquids change the pH balance (acidity) in your mouth and this interferes with nicotine absorption. If you need to drink one of these beverages, you should remove the gum, drink the liquid, and then rinse your mouth with water before reinserting the gum.

SIDE EFFECTS: If you chew the gum too fast, you may get effects similar to those experienced by people when they inhale a cigarette for the first time, or when they smoke a cigarette too fast. These effects include lightheadedness, nausea, vomiting, throat and mouth irritation, hiccups, and upset stomach. Most of these side effects can be controlled by chewing slowly. Other effects sometimes experienced, particularly during the first few days of using the gum, include sores in mouth, aching jaw, headache, heart palpitations, and more than the usual amount of saliva in the mouth. Please report any side effects to us.

NOTE: DO NOT SMOKE AT THE SAME TIME YOU ARE CHEWING THIS GUM.

If you accidentally swallow a piece of gum, you should not experience adverse effects. **If you do feel ill, call your doctor.** Overdosage could occur if many pieces are chewed simultaneously or in rapid succession. **In case of accidental overdose, or if a child chews or swallows more than one or two pieces of the gum, you should contact your physician or local poison control center immediately.**

Nicotine Transderm Patch (24 hour) Patient Information

HOW THE PATCH WORKS: The nicotine patch delivers nicotine to the body through the skin. The drug enters the body at a constant rate over a sustained period of time (24 hours). This patch has recently been shown to decrease the withdrawal symptoms of smoking, such as anxiety, nervousness, irritability, and poor concentration.

The patch is a useful alternative to nicotine gum for patients attempting to quit smoking. The nicotine patch is available in doses of 7 to 21 mg and is designed to be worn for 24 hours.

WHAT ABOUT SIDE EFFECTS? The nicotine patch is normally well tolerated. However, you should *not* smoke at the same time the patch is being used. The most common side effect is a local skin reaction under the patch. Although slight redness may occur initially, if severe redness with swelling persists 24 hours after removing the patch, you should stop using the patch and call your nurse or doctor. Patients with a history of skin problems may need to avoid using the patch.

HOW TO WEAR THE PATCH: The nicotine patch can be worn anywhere on the chest or outer upper arm. The skin should be hairless (or shaved) and free of irritation. The patch should not be worn under a skinfold or tight clothing. It is important to wash the skin and to carefully dry it before applying the patch. After 24 hours, remove the patch and apply a new patch to a *different* place on the chest or outer upper arm. Skin sites should not be reused for at least 7 days. You can wear the patch while bathing, swimming, exercising, and sweating. Apply patches at the same time each day so that you follow a schedule. It is important to observe any skin reactions. If severe redness and swelling do occur after removing the patch, call your nurse or doctor.

WHAT ABOUT DOSAGES? The patch is normally used daily for 8 to 12 weeks. A typical starting dosage is 14 to 21 mg for the first 4 weeks. The dosage is then decreased gradually to 7 mg. A schedule of doses will be given to you with your prescription. You will be asked to refill the prescription after 4 weeks.

WARNING TO FEMALE PARTICIPANTS: The patch does contain nicotine, which may cause fetal harm when used by pregnant women. Do not use the patch if you are pregnant or nursing.

REMEMBER: DO NOT SMOKE AT THE SAME TIME YOU ARE USING THE PATCH. Since nicotine is released through the patch, it should be kept away from children.

Self-Efficacy Questionnaire on Smoking

Instructions: These questions will help us to identify situations in which you are at risk of a relapse into smoking. Avoiding these situations can help you stay off cigarettes. Please answer every question even if it does not seem to apply to you personally.

Name _____ Date _____

Confidence Questionnaire

How confident are you that you can resist the urge to smoke in each of the following 14 situations?

Not at all confident			Slightly confident			Fairly confident			Very confident	
0%	10%	20%	30%	40%	50%	60%	70%	80%	90%	100%

Write number here

1. When you feel bored or depressed   _____

2. When you see others smoking   _____

3. When you want to relax or rest   _____

4. When you just want to sit back and enjoy a cigarette   _____

5. When you are watching TV   _____

6. When you are driving or riding in a car   _____

7. When you have finished a meal or snack   _____

8. When you feel frustrated, worried, upset, tense, nervous, angry, anxious, or annoyed   _____

9. When you want a snack, but don't want to gain weight   _____

10. When you need more energy or can't concentrate   _____

11. When someone offers you a cigarette   _____

12. When you are drinking coffee or tea   _____

13. When you are in a situation where alcohol is involved   _____

14. When you feel smoking is part of your self-image   _____

Telephone Interview for Patients Attempting to Quit Smoking

Name _____ Med Rec No _____

1. Have you used any tobacco product since we last talked? (Mark ''Yes'' if the patient has had even one puff or chew of any tobacco product.)

   ____ If no, continue to ''Not Smoking'' section below.

   N/Y If yes, proceed to #2.

2. Are you still smoking?

   ____ If no, continue to ''Lapse/Relapse'' section below.

   N/Y If yes, go to the ''Smoker'' section.

Not Smoking

1. Have you had any withdrawal symptoms?

   ____ If no, go to #4.

   N/Y If yes, continue to #2.

2. How severe have these withdrawal symptoms been?

   ____ 1 Not at all severe   2 Mildly severe   3 Moderately severe

   1-5   4 Severe   5 Very severe

3. How have you coped with these withdrawal symptoms or urges?

   _____

4. Are you using nicotine gum or the nicotine patch?

   ____ If no, go to #6.

   N/Y If yes, continue to #5.

5. How much nicotine are you using daily?

   ____ pieces of gum

   ____ mg of nicotine patch

6. How confident are you that you will not start smoking again?

   ____ (0 = no confidence; 100 = total confidence)

If confidence is less than 70%, use problem-solving techniques to help the patient understand why this is the case, and ask the patient to call you if urges to smoke are causing difficulty. Encourage the patient to find another support person to contact during these difficult times. Congratulate the patient on his or her success and remind him or her that you will be calling again soon.

Lapse/Relapse

1. When did you begin smoking?

   ____ /____ /____ mo/day/yr

2. Where were you when you started smoking?

   _____

3. What triggered your relapse? (Enter the most important item.)

   ____ 1 Emotions
        2 Alcohol
        3 A situation that you associate with smoking
        4 Peer pressure
        5 Stress
        6 Withdrawal symptoms
        7 Wanting to test yourself

4. How did you cope with this relapse? (Review how the patient coped with the relapse situation here.)

   _____

5. On a scale of 1 to 5, with 5 being very strong, how strong was your urge to smoke at that time?

   ____ 1 Not at all severe   2 Mildly severe   3 Moderately severe
   1-5   4 Severe   5 Very severe

6. Have you smoked a puff or more of a cigarette, cigar, cigarello, or pipeful of tobacco during the past five consecutive days?

   ____ No
   N/Y Yes

7. Have you been given a prescription for nicotine gum or the nicotine patch?

   ____ If no, go to #7
   N/Y If yes, continue to #8

8. How much are you using daily?
   ____ pieces of gum
   ____ mg of nicotine patch

9. On a scale of 1 to 7, how would you rate your intention to stay off cigarettes or other tobacco products?

   ____ 1 Definitely no   2 Probably no   3 Possibly no
   1-7   4 Maybe   5 Possibly yes
         6 Probably yes   7 Definitely yes

10. How confident are you that you will not start smoking again?

   ____ (0 = no confidence; 100 = total confidence)

If intention is less than 5 or confidence is less than 70%, use problem-solving techniques to help the patient understand why this is the case. Make sure you have reviewed the relapse situation, and discuss what the patient would do if faced with another temptation. Urge the patient to identify a support person to contact during difficult times.

11. Do you want a prescription for nicotine gum or the nicotine patch now?

_____

N/Y

Congratulate the patient for his or her success in getting back on track, and remind him or her that you will be calling again at the next scheduled time.

Smoker

If questions 1 to 5 have been completed on a previous call, go to #6. If they have not, complete them now.

1. When did you begin smoking?

___ /___ /___ mo/day/yr

2. Where were you when you started smoking?

_____

3. What triggered your relapse? (Enter the most important item.)

_____ 1 Emotions
    2 Alcohol
    3 A situation that you associate with smoking
    4 Peer pressure
    5 Stress
    6 Withdrawal symptoms
    7 Wanting to test yourself

4. How did you cope with this relapse? (Review how the patient coped with the relapse situation here.)

_____

5. On a scale of 1 to 5, with 5 being very strong, how strong was your urge to smoke at that time?

_____ 1 Not at all severe   2 Mildly severe   3 Moderately severe
1-5   4 Severe   5 Very severe

6. Are you using nicotine gum or the nicotine patch?

_____

N/Y

7. How much nicotine are you using daily?

_____ pieces of gum
_____ mg of nicotine patch

8. What is the average number of cigarettes per day (or cigars, pipes, or cigar-ellos) that you have smoked since we last talked?

     _____ # of cigarettes

9. On a scale of 1 to 7, how would you rate your intention to stay off cigarettes or other tobacco products?

     _____ 1 Definitely no   2 Probably no   3 Possibly no
     1-7   4 Maybe   5 Possibly yes
            6 Probably yes   7 Definitely yes

10. How confident are you that you can stop smoking now?

     _____ (0 = no confidence; 100 = total confidence)

If intention is less than 5 or confidence is less than 70%, use problem-solving techniques to help the patient understand why this is the case. Make sure you have reviewed the relapse situation, and discuss what the patient would do if faced with another temptation. Urge the patient to identify a support person to contact during difficult times.

11. Are you willing to quit now?

     _____ If no, encourage the patient to again think seriously about quitting.
     N/Y   End call.
            If yes, continue to #12.

If patient has not had an extra visit, ask him or her to come in within 48 hours if possible (only one relapse visit is permitted). Schedule a visit and ask the patient if he or she is experiencing any contraindications to nicotine gum. If patient is unwilling to come in for a visit, ask if you can set another quit date over the telephone. State that you'll call patient at next scheduled time.

12. Can we schedule a visit within the next 48 hours?

     _____ If no, schedule a quit date and tell the patient that you will call at the
     N/Y   next regularly scheduled time.
            If yes, schedule a visit now. Enter the date and time below.

13. Relapse visit date   Time

     ___ /___ /___   ___:___

14. Quit date   Time

     ___ /___ /___   ___:___

15. Date of post-relapse call   Time

     ___ /___ /___   ___:___

16. Do you want a prescription for nicotine gum or the nicotine patch now?

     ____
     N/Y

Chapter 9

Adherence to Medications

A ny discussion of lifestyle modification for coronary heart disease patients must take into account the importance of maintaining medications. These medications often cause unpleasant side effects, and many must be taken for life. Medications are used to control hypertension, to manage lipids, to influence prognosis, to control arrhythmias, to alter clotting, and to prevent or control angina. It is not uncommon for coronary patients to be taking 4 to 8 medications per day. Indeed, in the MULTIFIT program, the average patient was prescribed 4 to 5 medications per day in the year following infarction. In this chapter we will discuss how health care professionals can assist patients with medication adherence, including maintenance, and we will identify ways to assess non-adherence.

Adherence to all medications is a significant problem, not only for the coronary population, but for the American public in general. Data from the National Pharmaceutical Council indicates that only 61% of patients who start taking antihypertensive medications are still taking them after 12 months (Houston Miller, Stoy, & Thomas, 1994). Studies conducted in the elderly population find nonadherence levels of 40% or more when complex schedules are involved (Cooper, Love, & Raffoul, 1982; Leirer, Morrow, Pariante, & Sheikh, 1988). It is known that the more complex the regimen (i.e., the greater number of drugs that must be taken) the greater the likelihood of nonadherence.

Why does adherence appear to be such a problem for patients? There are many barriers associated with a lack of adherence, including poor communication between the health care provider and the patient; patients' beliefs, such as denial of illness, nonacceptance of a chronic disease, belief that a therapy will or will not work, and fear or misunderstanding of side effects; and the complexity of the drug regimen (Burgess, 1989; Clepper, 1992). Other factors which may compromise medication therapy after initiation include lifestyle changes (moving, marriage, job changes), psychological distress, lack of social support, and irregular schedules. All of these factors must be carefully considered when dealing with nonadherence.

Because many of the medications prescribed for coronary heart disease can have an effect on prognosis (i.e., antiplatelet agents, lipid-lowering medications, beta blockers, antihypertensive drugs, etc.), the coronary patient must develop an adequate system for managing medications. The first step in this process is education about the appropriate administration of a drug. The rehabilitation setting also provides an opportunity for ongoing assessment of medication taking, reinforcement, problem solving, and feedback based on changes in physiological indicators such as blood pressure, lipoproteins, and incidence of angina.

Initiating Medication Therapy

The way in which medication therapy is initiated can have a major influence on the patient's success in maintaining the medication schedule. While in most cases the health care professionals who initiate medication therapy are physicians, rehabilitation specialists can support the process with ongoing education and problem solving in the early phases of medication taking. This may require close coordination with the physician. As suggested in the literature on anti-hypertensive regimens, there are three key strategies that are useful in the process of educating patients about their regimens. These include (1) correcting any misconceptions the patient may have about a regimen, (2) adjusting the medication to the patient's lifestyle, and (3) enhancing support from family members (U.S. Department of Health and Human Services, 1987).

Some patients have no idea why a medication has been prescribed, how long they are to take a medication, or the goals of therapy. Moreover, they may hear from another friend or family member the horror stories of "Aunt Emma's experience in taking the same medication." For these reasons, it is important to discuss the potential hazards of self-adjusting a medication regimen or discontinuing a drug.

Adjusting a medication to the patient's lifestyle may also help ensure adherence. The health care professional should express a willingness to modify the dosage or frequency of a medication to solve practical problems that may make the regimen incompatible with the patient's lifestyle. Rehabilitation specialists working in collaboration with physicians often help in the process of readjusting the timing of medications so as to optimize the effect of the medication in controlling blood pressure or glucose in the case of hypertensive or diabetic patients.

Family members can be extremely helpful in providing encouragement, supporting the patient's adherence to medication, and reminding the patient about the specifics of a regimen. Simply identifying one influential person within the household who can remind the patient about their medications until it becomes "routine" may be helpful in the early stages of initiation.

In the MULTIFIT program, nurses initiate medication therapy for patients needing lipid-lowering medications. They utilize the following 6-step approach to educate the patient:

1. Inquire about past experiences the patient has had in taking lipid-lowering medications.
2. Write an appropriate administration schedule on the patient's "Medication Information Sheet" (for an example see p. 111). Ask the patient to post this on his or her refrigerator.

3. Ask the patient to repeat the instructions they have been given for administering their medication. Clarify any misinformation.
4. Ascertain factors which may contribute to decreased adherence (e.g., travel, illness, stressors).
5. Ask the patient to use a medication calendar for the first month of therapy.
6. Formalize your willingness to work with the patient by signing a written agreement. Tell the patient you will telephone them in one week about their medication(s). Determine a method to help the patient remember to take a medication. Read the "Medication Information Sheet" about the specific drug.

Patients leave the rehabilitation setting with information materials about the specific drug they are to begin taking, including a titration schedule if necessary, and a medication calendar which is to be used for one month and mailed back to the nurse. In their initial 30-minute session, patients are taught to differentiate side effects which are normal but short-term, those that are longer-term but should dissipate with time, and those which require immediate attention through a telephone call. Patients are encouraged to telephone when they have problems with the administration of a drug or with side effects, especially in the first week of use of the medication. Nurses also work very closely with patients to develop a plan for refilling medications one week prior to essential refills.

Maintenance of Medication Regimens

There are two problems, often associated with taking medications, that may be cited as reasons for low adherence rates. Forgetting to take a medication and dose omissions account for up to 80% of the deviations from a prescription (Cramer et al., 1989; Kass, Gordon, Morley, Meltzer, & Goldberg, 1987; Rudd, Ahmed, Zachary, Barton, & Bonduelle, 1990). Forgetting to take a medication occurs intermittently without an obvious pattern. However, it is also known that patients initiate "drug holidays," or days without drug use, which appear to be related to interruptions in daily schedules such as holidays or weekends. These holidays may lead to hospital admissions (Vinson, Rich, Sperry, Shah, & McNamara, 1990). In addition, although side effects are not always cited as a major reason for lapsing with medications (Rudd & Marshall, 1985), patients often attempt to titrate their pills to minimize drug reactions (DiTullio et al., 1988) and to increase their sense of autonomy (Conrad, 1985).

Several behavioral strategies can be employed to help improve the likelihood that a patient will maintain the medication regimen. Most often these include prompting, self-monitoring, and, to a lesser extent, relapse prevention training.

Prompting

Prompting the behavior is known to increase adherence. In the MULTIFIT program, each patient is asked to identify a prompt which will serve as a cue for medication taking. Such prompts include posting a medication sheet on the refrigerator, using medication dispensers which are placed on the kitchen table, or using a wristwatch with a timer as a reminder to take a medication. For elderly patients or those with multiple medications, using a device that has compartments labeled for the days of the week is helpful as a reminder to take the appropriate medications.

Self-Monitoring

Self-monitoring is a second behavioral method that may help patients adhere to their regimens. If patients are asked to record when they take a medication for the first month or two after initiation, they may begin to identify periods when they are taking doses later than prescribed or periods when they are likely to forget a dose. Such monitoring can help the patient and the rehabilitation specialist develop strategies for overcoming some of the difficulties associated with missed doses or irregular schedules. In the MULTIFIT program, self-monitoring is undertaken through the use of medication calendars for 1 month after the patient initiates a new medication.

Relapse Prevention

Relapse prevention training is most commonly used to treat addictive behaviors. However, it may be useful in preventing medication lapses as well. The patient and health care professional should identify and prepare for situations in which taking medications may be problematic. One of the most common times in which a patient forgets to take a medication is during a vacation. Planning ahead by altering schedules and increasing the use of reminders during these times may improve adherence.

Managing Side Effects

Side effects have been implicated as a reason for nonadherence to medication regimens (Kern & Baile, 1986; Moore, 1988). However, in some reviews (DiMatteo & DiNicola, 1982), side effects have not been shown to heavily influence adherence to a medication. In these studies, the presence of side effects was similar for nonadherers and adherers (DiMatteo & DiNicola, 1982). In the MULTIFIT program, although as many as 40% of patients reported side effects of lipid-lowering medications, fewer than 6% required a change in medication therapies (Miller et al., 1991). Side effects must be considered a problem and should be discussed in an effort to identify methods to minimize them. We suggest a simple approach to help the patient in this process:

1. Clarify information about side effects (e.g., are they attributable to a drug, are they chronic, are they a mask for other reasons of noncompliance).

2. Help the patient develop strategies for managing side effects (e.g., use hygienic measures, determine if doses can be reduced, change administration schedules).
3. Determine the patient's level of motivation to continue taking a medication (e.g., ascertain the patient's willingness to continue taking the medication, consider identifying new drugs which may have fewer side effects).

Although many side effects are not serious and can be managed using problem-solving strategies, the more serious effects must be dealt with promptly, and medications must be stopped if indicated. Rehabilitation specialists can play a key role in the process of assessing nonadherence.

Follow-Up Assessment of Nonadherence

Approximately 50 to 60% of patients will comply in taking their medications and will adhere to recommended schedules. At the other extreme, 5 to 10% of patients will be nonadherent and will not take medications appropriately under any circumstances. Finally, 30 to 40% of patients are known as ''partial adherers;'' they accept that they must take their medications, but do so inappropriately and inconsistently (Rudd, 1992). In order to detect and assist the partial adherers, it is important to ask all patients in follow-up how they are managing their medications.

Half of all patients who are nonadherent to medications can be identified simply by posing specific, nonthreatening questions or statements to the patient (Cohen, 1985). Providing statements which are confrontive but also nonthreatening may help patients realize the problem of nonadherence and may lead to a problem-solving approach to change. Below is a list of questions which can be used during telephone calls or in the rehabilitation setting to help assess problems and to estimate the patient's likelihood of nonadherence.

"Can you describe for me when and how you take your medication each morning?"

"Do you take your medication at different times on the weekends?"

"How many doses of medication do you think you have missed in the past week?"

"Many patients find it difficult to take their medications on a regular basis. I know I do. Do you ever miss or forget to take your medications?"

"When you feel better, do you sometimes stop taking your medication?"

"Can you tell me how you remember to take your medication when you travel (during times of high stress, etc.)?"

"Sometimes, if you feel worse when you take a medication, do you stop taking it?"

"Do you anticipate any changes in your lifestyle over the next couple of months that might interfere with your taking your medication?"

In addition to direct confrontation or probing to detect problems with medication taking, the health care professional can use various techniques to elicit responses in which patients reveal feelings and attitudes or beliefs about a specific treatment regimen. This is done using such statements as, "You seem discouraged about taking your medications," or "You seem uncomfortable about discussing your medications." Such questions can help the health care professional uncover problems with motivation. Important additional information may be obtained by asking patients about the location of their medications and about the cues they use as reminders.

One should be alert to the fact that, in addition to forgetting to take a medication and side effects, there may be other reasons for lack of adherence. Situations that may affect adherence to other medication regimes include travel, life stressors, lack of motivation, illnesses and hospitalization, inadequate social support, and feeling tired and bored with a regimen. It is helpful to ascertain if any of these situations is problematic for a patient.

Outcome Goals for Medication Taking

The goal of measuring outcomes is to determine the patient's level of adherence to medication regimens and to monitor responses to drug therapy based on adherence. While there are many ways to monitor medication adherence, such as patient diaries, pill counts, mechanical monitors, and clinician estimates, interviews with patients may be the most effective method (Cohen, 1985). Interviews have shown a correlation of 0.75 with pill counts in some studies (Craig, 1985). Important information about the patient's level of adherence can be obtained using simple questions about daily dosage administration, timing, and side effects, and by developing scenarios to determine when a patient may fail to take a medication. If the level of adherence is less than prescribed, the health care professional should seek to identify the important barriers to medication adherence. Emphasis should be placed on problem solving to increase adherence, or patients should be referred to their personal physicians so that appropriate medication adjustments can be made.

Summary

The patient with coronary heart disease is often prescribed multiple medications following a CHD event. The patient's likelihood of adherence to medication regimens can be improved by providing systematic education about the initiation of new medications and by helping the patient to develop strategies for maintenance. Simple questions can be used to assess side effects and potential problems of nonadherence and to determine if barriers to taking specific medications can be overcome.

Medication Information Sheet

Patient Information
on Bile Acid Binding Resins
Cholestyramine (Questran™)
and Colestipol (Colestid™)

WHAT DO THEY DO? Bile acid binding resins like Cholestyramine (Questran™) and colestipol (Colestid™) work in the intestines by binding bile as it leaves the gall bladder. These resins decrease the absorption of fat and cholesterol in the intestine and also decrease production of cholesterol in the liver. These medications are not absorbed into the bloodstream.

WHAT DO THEY LOOK LIKE? Cholestyramine and colestipol come in powder form in bulk containers (cans or bottles) or in packets (one scoop = one packet). A full dose is 4 to 6 scoops or packets per day. These medicines must always be mixed with liquids or "watery" foods.

HOW SHOULD I TAKE THEM? It is important to take these medications properly and to start slowly. (See tips below.) The daily dose is divided between a morning and an evening dose. The drug works best when taken 20 to 30 minutes before the morning or evening meal. These medications can be mixed with water (2 to 4 oz) or, more effectively, with fruit juices or Tang™ to improve the taste and texture. A day's supply can be mixed in a blender and stored in the refrigerator. You can also sprinkle the medication over applesauce or put it in yogurt, cereal, or fruit if you cannot tolerate it plain.

WHAT ABOUT SIDE EFFECTS? The most common side effects are described below:

- **Constipation**. To avoid constipation, you should drink plenty of water (four 8-oz glasses unless on fluid restriction), get regular exercise, increase your dietary fiber (fruits, vegetables, whole grains, and bran) or use Metamucil™ or Miller's Bran™ according to package directions.
- **Gas, bloating, stomach cramps**. These side effects usually go away after using the resin for 1 to 2 weeks. If they persist, try mixing the medication with another liquid, or use nonconstipating medications such as Simethicone™, Riopan Plus™, or Mylanta™.
- **Rare side effects**. The following side effects, which are relatively rare, should be reported to your doctor or nurse: severe stomach pains with nausea/vomiting, black stools, sudden weight loss.

ARE THERE ANY SPECIAL PRECAUTIONS? Resins may interfere with the absorption of other medications, including thyroid pills, digoxin, diuretics, beta blocking agents, coumadin, tetracycline, penicillin G, and possibly fat-soluble vitamins (A, D, E, and K). **For this reason, you should take these other medications either 1 hour before or 4 to 6 hours after taking cholestyramine or colestipol.** People with active bowel disease or active or recent ulcer should not take resins. Some people with severe constipation or hemorrhoids might also need to avoid resins.

TIPS FOR TAKING RESINS

- Start "slow and low." Start with one packet or scoop daily and gradually increase the dose. (See your schedule below.)
- If constipation is a problem, *don't* stop taking the drug. Call your nurse.
- Do not miss a dose because you missed a meal. Take your dose even if you don't eat.
- Bowel gas is not uncommon. A medication called Simethicone™, which can be purchased at your local pharmacy, can help break up gas bubbles.
- Drink at least four 8-oz glasses of fluids daily unless you are on fluid restriction. If you cannot tolerate Metamucil™, or constipation is severe, try wheat bran.

WHAT IS MY PRESCRIPTION? You should take your cholestyramine or colestipol based on this schedule:

Date(s)		Morning dose	Evening dose
_____	(Days)	_____	_____
_____	(Days)	_____	_____
_____	(Days)	_____	_____
_____	(Days)	_____	_____
_____	(Days)	_____	_____
_____	(Days)	_____	_____

Directions for Preparing Bile Acid Binding Resins

The medication may be mixed with water, another liquid, or a fruit juice with high fluid content. The scoop of medication should be sprinkled on top of 4 to 6 fluid ounces of liquid. Note: the medication should be allowed to float on top of the liquid for 1 to 2 minutes, then stir well. The drug will not completely dissolve because it is not water soluble. A larger amount of fluid may be used if desired. Use cold to lukewarm liquids and a wide mouth glass, which will allow the medication to absorb water and dissolve better.

The medication can also be mixed in a shaker or blender. Similarly, float the medication on top of 4 to 6 ounces of fluid for 1 to 2 minutes. Shake or blend until the drug is suspended; this usually takes about 30 seconds.

Tests show that mixing the drug prior to drinking is more acceptable than mixing the total number of scoops and allowing it to stand for several hours.

However, preparing a day's supply at one time may be more convenient. This must be kept in a refrigerator or thermos, and should be kept no longer than 24 hours. The mixture should be shaken well before each dosage is taken.

For a single day's supply, place 24 to 36 ounces of liquid in a container and sprinkle the entire day's supply (2 to 6 scoops) on the surface of the liquid. Allow the medication to stand for several minutes, then stir well or blend.

DRUG MIXTURES

Water: Using water is the most common and easiest way of preparing the drug. Questran™ may turn the water yellowish and it will taste like a mild Tang™ drink.

Orange juice: Use full strength or dilute with equal parts of water and orange juice.

V-8 Juice: The medication produces a mild flavor change.

Coke: A foam will form when the medication is mixed with coke.

Sprite or Gingerale: When the medication is mixed with soda, it will taste like lemon-lime and may turn the liquid yellow.

Beef broth: Warm the broth first, then add the powder.

Tang™, Grapefruit juice: Is perhaps most tasty (it tastes like orange).

Banana Shake:
1 banana
1/2 cup skim milk
1-3 scoops of drug

Beat in blender

Vanilla Shake:
1/2 cup vanilla-flavored Weight Watchers™ frozen dessert
1-3 scoops of drug

Beat in blender

Banana "Daiquiri":
1 banana
1 cup crushed ice
1-3 scoops of drug

Beat in blender

Orange Shake:
1/2 cup orange sherbet
1/2 cup skim milk
1-3 scoops of drug

Beat in blender

References

Adler, E. (1993). *Everyone's guide to successful publications: How to produce powerful brochures, newsletters, flyers, and business communications.* Berkeley: Peachpit Press.

Adsett, C.A., & Bruhn, J.G. (1968). Short-term group psychotherapy for post-myocardial infarction patients and their wives. *Canadian Medical Association Journal,* **99,** 577-584.

Agras, W.S., Taylor, C.B., Kraemer, H.C., Southam, M.A., & Schneider, J.A. (1987). Relaxation training for essential hypertension at the worksite: II. The poorly controlled hypertensive. *Psychosomatic Medicine,* **49,** 264-273.

Andrew, G.M., Oldridge, N.B., & Parker, J.O. (1981). Reasons for dropout from exercise programs in post-coronary patients. *Medicine and Science in Sports and Exercise,* **13,** 164-168.

Bandura, A. (1986*). Social foundations of thought and action: A social cognitive theory.* Englewood Cliffs, NJ: Prentice Hall.

Bandura, A. (1977). *Social Learning Theory.* Englewood Cliffs, NJ: Prentice Hall.

Barbarowicz, P., Nelson, M., DeBusk, R.F., & Haskell, W.L. (1980). A comparison of in-hospital education approaches for coronary bypasss patients. *Heart and Lung,* **9,** 127-133.

Barefoot, J.C., Dahlstrom W.G., & Williams R.B. (1983). Hostility, CHD incidence, and total mortality: A 25-year follow-up study of 255 physicians. *Psychosomatic Medicine,* **45,** 59-63.

Barry, J., Mead, K., Nabel, E., Rocco, M.B., Campbell, S., Fenton, T., Mudge, G.H. Jr., & Selwyn, A.P. (1989). Effect of smoking on the activity of ischemic heart disease. *Journal of the American Medical Association,* **261,** 398-402.

Beck, A.T., Ward, C.H., Mendelson, M., Mock, J., & Erbaugh, J. (1961). An inventory for measuring depression. *Archives of General Psychiatry,* **4,** 561-571.

Becker, M.H. (1974). The Health Belief Model and personal health behavior. *Health Education Monographs,* **2,** 236-508.

Beckie, T. (1989). A supportive-educative telephone program: Impact on knowledge and anxiety after coronary artery bypass graft surgery. *Heart and Lung,* **18,** 46-55.

Benight, C.C., & Taylor, C.B. (1994). The effects of exercise on improving anxiety, depression, emotional well-being and elements of Type A behavior. In D.L. Elliot & L. Goldberg (Eds.), *Exercise as Medical Therapy* (pp. 319-332). Philadelphia: F.A. Davis.

Benowitz, N.L. (1988). Drug therapy: Pharmacologic aspects of cigarette smoking and nicotine addiction. *New England Journal of Medicine,* **319,** 1318-1330.

Benson, H. (1976). *The Relaxation Response.* Boston: G.K. Hall.

116   References

Benson, H., Beary, J.F., & Carol, M.P. (1974). The Relaxation Response. *Psychiatry*, **37** (1), 37-46.

Blankenhorn, D.H., Azen, S.P., Kransch, D.M., Mack, W.J., Cashin-Hemphill, L., Hodis, H.N., DeBoer, L.W., Mahrer, P.R., Masteller, M.J., & Vailas, L.I. (1993). Coronary angiographic changes with Lovastatin therapy: The Monitored Atherosclerosis Study (MARS). *Annals of Internal Medicine*, **119**, 969-976.

Blankenhorn, D.H., Nessim, S.A., Johnson, R.L., Sanmarco, M.E., Azen, S.P., & Cashin-Hemphill, L. (1987). Beneficial effects of combined colestipol-niacin therapy on coronary atherosclerosis and coronary venous bypass grafts. *Journal of the American Medical Association*, **257**, 3233-3240.

Block, G. (1982). A review of validations of dietary assessment methods. *American Journal of Epidemiology*, **115**, 492-505.

Burgess, M.M. (1989). Ethical and economic aspects of noncompliance and overtreatment. *Canadian Medical Association Journal*, **141**, 777-780.

Burkett, P.A., Rectanus, E.F., & Bultena, K. (1990). Compliance to a Phase III exercise program [Abstract]. *Journal of Cardiopulmonary Rehabilitation*, **10**, 381.

Burling, T.A., Singleton, E.G., Bigelow, G.E., Baile, W.F., & Gottlieb, S.H. (1984). Smoking following myocardial infarction: A critical review of the literature. *Health Psychology*, **3**, 83-96.

Burnett, K.F., Magel, P.E., Harrington, S., & Taylor, C.B. (1989). Computer-assisted behavioral health counseling for high school students. *Journal of Counseling Psychology*, **36**, 1-5.

Burnett, K., Taylor, C.B., & Agras, W.S. (1985). Ambulatory computer-assisted therapy for obesity: A new frontier for behavior therapy. *Journal of Consulting and Clinical Psychology*. **53**, 698-703.

Burnett, K.F., Taylor, C.B., & Agras, W.S. (1992). Ambulatory computer-assisted behavior therapy for obesity: An empirical model for examining behavioral correlates of treatment outcome. *Computers in Human Behavior*, **8**, 239-248.

Burt, A., Thornley, P., Illingworth, D., White, P., Shaw, T.R., & Turner, R. (1974). Stopping smoking after myocardial infarction. *Lancet*, **1** (852), 304-306.

Case, R.B., Moss, A.J., Case, N., McDermott, M., & Eberly, S. (1992). Living alone after myocardial infarction: Impact on prognosis. *Journal of the American Medical Association*, **267**, 515-519.

Choudhary, S., Jackson, P., Katan, M.B., Marenah, C.B., Cortese, C., Miller, N.E., & Lewis, B. (1984). A multifactorial diet in the management of hyperlipidemia. *Atherosclerosis*, **50**, 93-103.

Clark, E., DeBusk, R.F., Johansson, M., Hyman, D., & Corsetto, C. (1988). Telephone-mediated dietary intervention for hypercholesterolemia. *First National Cholesterol Conference, Proceedings*, 107.

Clepper, I. (1992). Noncompliance, the invisible epidemic. *Drug Topics*.

Cohen, S., Kamarck, T., & Mermelstein, R. (1983). A global measure of perceived stress. *Journal of Health and Social Behavior*, **24**, 385-396.

Cohen, S.J. (1985). Improving patients' compliance with anti-hypertensive regimens. *Comprehensive Therapy*, **11**, 18-21.

Comoss, P.M. (1992). Education of the coronary patient and family: Principles and practice. In N.K. Wenger & H.K. Hellerstein (Eds.), *Rehabilitation of the Coronary Patient* (3rd ed., pp. 439-460). New York: Churchill Livingstone.

Condiotte, M.M., & Lichtenstein, E. (1981). Self-efficacy and relapse in smoking cessation programs. *Journal of Consulting Clinical Psychology*, **49**, 648-658.

Connor, S.L., Gustafson, J.R., Sexton, G., Becker, N., Artaud-Wild, S., & Connor, W.E. (1992). The Diet Habit Survey: A new method of dietary assessment that relates to plasma cholesterol changes. *Journal of the American Dietetic Association*, **92**(1), 41-47.

Conrad, P. (1985). The meaning of medications: Another look at compliance. *Social Science and Medicine*, **20**, 29-37.

Cooper, J.K., Love, D.W., & Raffoul, P.R. (1982). Intentional prescription non-adherence (noncompliance) by the elderly. *Journal of American Geriatric Society*, **30**, 329-333.

Craig, H.M. (1985). Accuracy of indirect methods of medication compliance in hypertension. *Research in Nursing and Health*, **8**, 61-66.

Cramer, J.A., Mattson, R.H., Prevey, M.I., Prevey, M.L., Scheyer, R.D., & Ouellette, V.L. (1989). How often is medication taken as prescribed? A novel assessment technique. *Journal of the American Medical Association*, **261**, 3273-3277.

Cummings, S., & Richard, R. (1988). Optimum cutoff points for biochemical validation of smoking status. *American Journal of Public Health*, **78**, 574-575.

Daly, L.E., Graham, I.M., Hickey, N., & Mulcahy, R. (1985). Does stopping smoking delay onset of angina after myocardial infarction? *British Medical Journal Clinical Research Education*, **291**, 935-937.

Deanfield, J., Wright, C., Krikler, S., Ribeiro, P., & Fox, K. (1984). Cigarette smoking and treatment of angina with propranolol, atenolol and nifedipine. *New England Journal of Medicine*, **310**, 951-954.

DeBusk, R.F., Haskell, W.L., Miller, N.H., Berra, K., Taylor, C.B., Berger, W.E. III, & Lew, H. (1985). Medically directed at-home rehabilitation soon after clinically uncomplicated myocardial infarction: A new model for patient care. *American Journal of Cardiology*, **55**, 251-257.

DeBusk, R.F., Houston, N., Haskell, W., Parker, M., & Fry, G. (1979). Exercise training soon after myocardial infarction. *American Journal of Cardiology*, **44**, 1223-1229.

DeBusk, R.F., Miller, N.H., Superko, H.R., Dennis, C.A., Thomas, R.J., Lew, H.T., Berger, W.E. III, Heller, R.S., Rompf, J., Gee, D., Kraemer, H.C., Bandura, A., Ghandour, G., Clark, M., Fisher, L., & Taylor, C.B. (1994). A case-management system for coronary risk factor modification after acute myocardial infarction. *Annals of Internal Medicine*, **120** (9), 721-729.

Dembroski, T.M., MacDougall, J.M., Costa, P.T., & Grandits, G.A. (1989). Components of hostility as predictors of sudden death and myocardial infarction in the Multiple Risk Factor Intervention Trial. *Psychosomatic Medicine*, **51**, 514-522.

DiMatteo, M.R., & DiNicola, D.D. (1982). *Achieving patient compliance: The psychology of the medical practitioner's role.* Elmsford, NY: Pergammon Press.

Dishman, R.K., & Gettman, L.R. (1980). Psychobiological influences on exercise adherence. *Journal of Sports Psychology,* 2, 295-310.

Dishman, R.K., & Steinhardt, M. (1988). Reliability and concurrent validity for a seven-day recall of physical activity in college students. *Medicine and Science in Sports and Exercise,* 20, 14-25.

DiTullio, N., Alli, C., Avanzini, F., Bettelli, G., Colombo, F., Devoto, M.A., Marchioli, R., Mariotti, G., Radice, M., & Taioli, E. (1988). Prevalence of symptoms generally attributable to hypertension or its treatment: Study on blood pressure in elderly outpatients. (SPAA) *Journal of Hypertension,* 6 (Suppl.), S87-S90.

Eaker, E.D. (1989). Psychosocial factors in the epidemiology of coronary heart disease in women. *Psychiatric Clinics of North America,* 12, 167-173.

Ewart, C.K., Taylor, C.B., Reese, L.B., & DeBusk, R.F. (1983). Effects of early postmyocardial infarction exercise testing on self-perception and subsequent physical activity. *American Journal of Cardiology,* 51, 1076-1080.

Ewing, J.A. (1984). Detecting alcoholism: The CAGE Questionnaire. *Journal of the American Medical Association,* 252, 1905-1907.

Fagerström, K.O. (1978). Measuring degree of physical dependence to tobacco smoking with reference to individualization of treatment. *Addictive Behaviors,* 3, 235-241.

Farquhar, J.W., Fortmann, S.P., Flora, J.A., Taylor, C.B., Haskell, W.L., Williams, P.T., Maccoby, N., & Wood, P.D. (1990). The Stanford Five-City Project: Effects of community-wide education on cardiovascular disease risk factors. *Journal of the American Medical Association,* 264, 359-365.

Fortmann, S.P., Taylor, C.B., Flora, J.A., & Winkleby, M.A. (1993). Effect of community health education on plasma cholesterol levels in diet: The Stanford Five-City Project. *American Journal of Epidemiology,* 137, 1039-1055.

Frasure-Smith, N., & Prince, R.H. (1985). The Ischemic Heart Disease Life Stress Monitoring Program: Impact on mortality. *Psychosomatic Medicine,* 47, 431-445.

Frasure-Smith, N., & Prince, R.H. (1989). Long-term follow-up of the Ischemic Heart Disease Life Stress Monitoring Program. *Psychosomatic Medicine,* 51, 485-513.

Friedman, M., & Rosenman, R.H. (1959). Association of specific overt behavior pattern with blood and cardiovascular findings. *Journal of the American Medical Association,* 169, 1286-1296.

Friedman, M., Thoresen, C.E., Gill, J.J., Powell, L.H., Ulmer, D., Thompson, L., Price, V.A.,Rabin, D.D., Breall, W.S., & Dixon, T. (1984). Alteration of type A behavior and reduction in cardiac recurrences in postmyocardial infarction patients. *American Heart Journal*, **108**, 237-248.

Friedman, M., Thoresen, C.E., Gill, J.J., Ulmer, D., Powell, L.H., Price, V.A., Brown, B., Thompson, L., Rabin, D.D., & Breall, W.S. (1986). Alteration of Type A behavior and its effect on cardiac recurrences in post myocardial infarction patients: Summary results of the recurrent coronary prevention project. *American Heart Journal*, **112**, 653-665.

Galan, K.M., Deligonul, U., Kern, M.J., Chaitman, B.R., & Vandormael, M.G. (1988). Increased frequency of restenosis in patients continuing to smoke cigarettes after acute percutaneous transluminal angioplasty. *American Journal of Cardiology*, **6**, 260-263.

Garding, B.S., Kerr, J.C., & Bay, K. (1988). Effectiveness of a program of information and support for myocardial infarction patients recovering at home. *Heart and Lung*, **17**, 355-362.

Gellhorn, E. (1970). The emotions and the ergotropic trophotropic systems. *Psychologische Forschung*, **34** (1), 48-94.

Goldfried, M.R., & Davison, G.C. (1976). *Clinical behavior therapy*. New York: Holt Rinehart & Winston.

Gossard, D., Haskell, W.L., Taylor, C.B., Mueller, K.J., Adams, F.R., Chandler, M., Ahn, D.K., Miller, N.H., & DeBusk, R.F. (1986). Effects of low- and high-intensity home-based exercise training on functional capacity in healthy middle-aged men. *American Journal of Cardiology*, **57**, 446-449.

Gottlieb, A.M., Killen, J.D., Marlatt, G.A., & Taylor, C.B. (1987). Psychological and pharmacological influences in cigarette smoking: Effects of nicotine gum and expectancy on smoking withdrawal symptoms and relapse. *Journal of Counseling and Clinical Psychology*, **55**, 606-608.

Graham, L.E., Taylor, C.B., Hovell, M.F., & Siegel, W. (1983). Five-year follow-up to a behavioral weight loss program. *Journal of Consulting and Clinical Psychology*, **51**, 322-323.

Gruen, W. (1975). Effects of brief psychotherapy during the hospitalization period on the recovery process in heart attacks. *Journal of Consulting and Clinical Psychology*, **43**, 223-232.

Grunberg, N.E. (1982). The effects of nicotine and cigarette smoking on food consumption and taste preferences. *Addictive Behaviors*, **7**, 317-331.

Hagberg, J.M., Montain, S.J., Martin, W.H., & Ehsani, A.A. (1989). Effect of exercise training on 60-69 year old persons with essential hypertension. *American Journal of Cardiology*, **64**, 348-353.

Hall, S.M., Ginsberg, D., & Jones, R.T. (1986). Smoking cessation and weight gain. *Journal of Consulting and Clinical Psychology*, **54**, 342-346.

Hamilton, M. (1960). A rating scale for depression. *Journal of Neurology, Neurosurgery and Psychiatry*. **23**, 56-62.

Hartung, G.H., Squires, W.G., & Gotto, A.M. (1981). Effect of exercise training on plasma high-density lipoprotein cholesterol in coronary disease patients. *American Heart Journal*, **101**, 181-184.

Haskell, W.L., Alderman, E.L., Fair, J.M., Maron, D.J., Mackey, S.F., Superko, R., Williams, P.T., Johnstone, I.M., Champagne, M., Krauss, R.M., &

Farquhar, J.W. (1994). Effects of intensive multiple risk factor reduction on coronary atherosclerosis and clinical cardiac events in men and women with coronary artery disease (SCRIP). *Circulation*, **89**, 975-990.

Hecker, M.H., Chesney, M.A., Black, G.W., & Frautschi, N. (1988). Coronary-prone behaviors in the Western Collaborative Group Study. *Psychosomatic Medicine*, **50**, 153-164.

Hermanson, B., Omenn, G., Krommel, R., & Gersh, B.J. (1988). Beneficial six-year outcome of smoking cessation in older men and women with coronary artery disease: Results from the CASS registry. *New England Journal of Medicine*, **319**, 1365-1369.

Houston Miller, N.H., Stoy, D.B., & Thomas, T. (1994). *A Nurse's Guide to the Management of Cholesterol and Coronary Heart Disease* (Monograph). Princeton, NJ: Bristol-Myers Squibb Co.

Hunninghake, D.B., Stein, E.A., Dujonre, C.A., Harris, N.A., Feldman, E.B., Miller, V.T., Tobet, J.A., Laskahewski, P.M., Guitoer, E., Held, J., Taylor, A.M., Hopper, S., Leonard S.B., & Bewer, B.K. (1993). The efficacy of intensive dietary therapy alone or combined with Lorastatin in outpatients with hypercholesterolemia. *New England Journal of Medicine*, **328**, 1213-1219.

Hurt, R.D., Lauger, G.G., Offord, K.P., Kottke, T.E., & Dale, L.C. (1990). Nicotine-replacement therapy with use of a transdermal nicotine patch—a randomized double-blind placebo-controlled trial. *Mayo Clinic Proceedings*, **65**(12), 1529-1537.

Ibrahim, M.A., Feldman, J.G., & Sultz, H.A., et al. (1974). Management after myocardial infarction: A controlled trial of the effect of group psychotherapy. *International Journal of Psychiatric Medicine*, **5**, 253.

Ironson, G., Taylor, C.B., Boltwood, M., Bartzokis, T., Dennis, C., Chesney, M., Spitzer, S., & Segall, G. (1992). Effects of anger on left ventricular ejection fraction in coronary artery disease. *American Journal of Cardiology*, **70**, 281-285.

Jeffery, R.W. (1988). Dietary risk factors and their modification in cardiovascular disease. *Journal of Consulting and Clinical Psychology*, **56**, 350-357.

Juneau, M., Rogers, F., De Santos, V., Yee, M., Evans, A., Bohn, A., Haskell, W.L., Taylor, C.B., & DeBusk, R.F. (1987). Effectiveness of self-monitored home-based moderate-intensity exercise training in middle-aged men and women. *American Journal of Cardiology*, **60**, 66-70.

Kannel, W.B., Castelli, W.P., Gordon, T., & McNamara, P.M. (1971). Serum cholesterol, lipoproteins, and the risk of coronary heart disease. The Framingham Study. *Annals of Internal Medicine*, **74**, 1-12.

Kass, M.A., Gordon, M., Morley, R.E. Jr, Meltzer, D.W., & Goldberg, J.J. (1987). Compliance with topical timolol treatment. *American Journal of Ophthalmology*, **103**, 188-193.

Kendall, A., Levitsky, D., Strupp, B.J., & Lissner, L. (1991). Weight loss on a low-fat diet: consequence of imprecision of the control of food intake in humans. *American Journal of Clinical Nutrition*, **53**, 1124-1129.

Kern, D.A., & Baile, W.F. (1986). Patient compliance with medical advice. In L.R. Barker, J.R. Burton, & P.E. Zieve (Eds.), *Principles of ambulatory medicine* (2nd ed., pp. 41-57). Baltimore: Williams and Wilkins.

Kessler, L., Burns, B., Shapiro, S., Tischler, G.L., George, L.K., Hough, R.L., Bodison, D., & Miller, R.H. (1987). Psychiatric diagnoses of medical service users: Evidence from the Epidemiologic Catchment Area Program. *American Journal on Public Health*, **77**, 18-24.

Killen, J., Maccoby, N., & Taylor, C.B. (1984). Nicotine gum and self-regulation training in smoking relapse prevention. *Behavior Therapy*, **15**, 234-248.

King, A.C., & Frederiksen, L.W. (1984). Low-cost strategies for increasing exercise behavior. *Behavior Modification*, **8**, 3-21.

King, A.C., Haskell, W.L., Taylor, C.B., Kraemer, H.C., & DeBusk, R.F. (1991). Group- versus home-based exercise training in healthy older men and women. *Journal of the American Medical Association*, **266**, 1535-1542.

King, A.C., & Martin, J.E. (1993). Exercise Adherence and Maintenance. In J.L. Durstine (Ed.), *Resource manual for guidelines for exercise testing and prescription* (pp. 443-454). Philadelphia: Lea & Febiger.

King, A.C., Taylor, C.B., Haskell, W.L., & DeBusk, R.F. (1988). Strategies for increasing early adherence and long-term maintenance of home-based exercise training in healthy middle-aged men and women. *American Journal of Cardiology*, **61**, 628-632.

King, A.C., Taylor, C.B., Haskell, W.L., & DeBusk, R.F. (1989). Influence of regular exercise on psychological health: A randomized controlled trial of healthy, middle-aged adults. *Health Psychology*, **8**, 305-324.

Klatsky, A.L., Armstrong, M.A., & Friedman, G.D. (1992). Alcohol and mortality. *Annals of Internal Medicine*, **117**, 646-654.

Knapp, D.N. (1988). Behavioral management techniques and exercise promotion. In R.K. Dishman (Ed.), *Exercise adherence: Its impact on public health* (pp. 203-236). Champaign, IL: Human Kinetics.

Kris-Etherton, P.M., Krummel, D., Russell, M.E., Dreon, D., Mackey, S., Borchers, J., & Wood, P.D. (1988). The effect of diet on plasma lipids, lipoproteins, and coronary heart disease. *Journal of the American Dietetic Association*, **88**, 1373-1399.

LaRosa, J.C., Hunninghake, D., Bush, D., Criqui, M.H., Getz, G.S., Gotto, A.M. Jr., Grundy, S.M., Rakita, L., Robertson, R.M., & Weisfeldt, M.L. (1990). The cholesterol facts: A summary of the evidence relating dietary fats, serum cholesterol, and coronary heart disease. AHA Medical/Scientific Statement. *Circulation*, **81**, 1721-1733.

Leirer, V.O., Morrow, D.G., Pariante, G.M., & Sheikh, J.I. (1988). Elders non-adherence, its assessment and computer-assisted instruction for medication recall training. *Journal of American Geriatric Society*, **36**, 877-884.

Linn, L.S., & Yager, J. (1984). Recognition of depression and anxiety by primary physicians. *Psychosomatics*, **25**, 593-600.

The Lipid Research Clinic Coronary Primary Prevention Trial Results. (1984). I. Reduction in incidence of coronary heart disease. *Journal of the American Medical Association*, **251**, 351-364.

Maouad, J., Fernandez, F., Hebert, J.L., Zamani, K., Barrillon, A., & Gay, J. (1986). Cigarette smoking during coronary angiography: Differences on focal narrowing (spasm) of the coronary arteries in 13 patients with angina at rest and normal coronary angiograms. *Catheterization Cardiology Diagram*, **12**, 366-375.

Markiewicz, W., Houston, N., & DeBusk, R.F. (1977). Exercise testing soon after myocardial infarction. *Circulation*, **56**, 26-31.

Marlatt, G.A., & Gordon, J.R. (Eds.) (1985). *Relapse prevention: Maintenance strategies in the treatment of addiction*. New York: Guilford Press.

May, G.S., Eberlein, K.A., Furberg, C.D., Passamani, E.R., & DeMets, D.L. (1982). Secondary prevention after myocardial infarction: A review of long-term trials. *Progress in Cardiovascular Disease*, **24**, 331-362.

Meakin, C.J. (1992). Screening for depression in the medically ill: The future of paper and pencil tests. *British Journal of Psychiatry*, **160**, 212-216.

Miller, N.H., Haskell, W.L., Berra, K., & DeBusk, R.F. (1984). Home versus group exercise training for increasing functional capacity soon after myocardial infarction. *Circulation*, **70**, 645-649.

Miller, N.H., & Taylor, C.B. (1995). Behavior modification for risk factor reduction. In M. Pollack & D. Schmidt (Eds.), *Heart Disease and Rehabilitation* (3rd ed.). Champaign, IL: Human Kinetics.

Miller, N.H., Thomas, R.J., Superko, R.H., Ghandour, G., Taylor, C.B., & DeBusk R.F. (1991). Lipid-lowering therapy in post-MI patients: Efficacy of a nurse managed intervention. *Circulation*, **84** (Suppl. II), 328.

Miller, N.H., Wagner, E., & Rogers, P. (1988). Worksite based multifactorial risk intervention trial. *Journal of American College of Cardiology*, **11**, 207A.

Moore, M.A. (1988). Improving compliance with antihypertensive therapy. *American Family Physician*, **37**, 142-148.

Moos, R. (1988). Life stressors and coping resources influence health and well-being. *Psychological Assessment*, **4**, 133-158.

Mueller, K.R., Gossard, D., Adams, F.R., Taylor, C.B., Haskell, W.L., Kraemer, H.C., Ahn, D.K., Burnett, K., & DeBusk, R.F. (1986). Assessment of prescribed increases in physical activity: Application of a new method for microprocessor analysis of heart rate. *American Journal of Cardiology*, **57**, 441-445.

Multiple Risk Factor Intervention Trial Research Group. (1982). Multiple risk factor intervention trial: risk factor changes and mortality results. *Journal of the American Medical Association*, **248**, 1465-1477.

National Diet-Heart Study Research Group. (1968). The National Diet-Heart Study Final Report. *Circulation*, **37** (Suppl. I), I1-I428.

National Research Council, Committee on Diet and Health (1989). *Diet and health: Implications for reducing chronic disease risk*. Washington, DC: National Academy Press.

Nicklin, W.M. (1986). Postdischarge concerns of cardiac patients as presented via a telephone callback system. *Heart and Lung*, **15**, 268-272.

O'Connor, G.T., Buring, J.E., & Yusaf, S. (1989). An overview of randomized trials of rehabilitation with exercise after myocardial infarction. *Circulation*, **80**, 234-244.

Oldenburg, B., Perkins, R.J., & Andrews, G. (1985). Controlled trial of psychological intervention in myocardial infarction. *Journal of Consulting and Clinical Psychology*, **53**, 852-859.

Oldridge, N.B. (1982). Compliance and exercise in primary and secondary prevention of coronary heart disease: A review. *Preventive Medicine*, **11**, 56-70.

Oldridge, N.B. (1991). Compliance with cardiac rehabilitation services. *Journal of Cardiopulmonary Rehabilitation*, **11**, 116-127.

Oldridge, N.B., Guyalit, G.H., Fischer, M.E., & Rimm, A.A. (1988). Cardiac rehabilitation with exercise after myocardial infarction. *Journal of American Medical Asssociation*, **260**, 945-950.

Oldridge, N.B., & Jones, N.L. (1983). Improving patient compliance in cardiac rehabilitation: Effects of written agreement and self-monitoring. *Journal of Cardiopulmonary Rehabilitation*, **3**, 257-262.

Oldridge, N.B., Ragowski, B., & Gottleib, M. (1992). Use of outpatient cardiac rehabilitation services: Factors associated with attendance. *Journal of Cardiopulmonary Rehabilitation*, **12**, 25-31.

Ornish, D., Brown, S.E., Scherwitz, L.W., Billings, J.H., Armstrong, W.T., Ports, T.A., McLanahan, S.M., Kirkeeide, R.L., Brand, R.J., & Gould, K.L. (1990). Can lifestyle changes reverse coronary heart disease? The Lifestyle Heart Trial. *Lancet*, **336**, 129-133.

Petruzzello, S.J., Landers, D.M., Hatfield, B.D., Kubitz, K.A., & Salazar, W. (1991). A meta-analysis of the anxiety-reducing effects of acute and chronic exercise: Outcomes and mechanisms. *Sports Medicine*, **11**, 143-148.

Pitt, B., Mancini, G.B., Ellis, S.G., Rosman, H.S., Smith, S.A., & McGovern, M.E. (1994). Pravastatin Limitation of Atherosclerosis in the Coronary Arteries (PLAC I): Beneficial effects of Pravastatin on cardiovascular events. *Journal of the American College of Cardiology*, Abs 131A. (Special issue, 43rd Annual Scientific Sessions), 739-742.

Pozen, M.W., Stechmiller, J.A., Harris, W., Smith, S., Fried, D.D., & Voigt, G.C. (1977). A nurse rehabilitator's impact on patients with myocardial infarction. *Medical Care*, **15**, 830-837.

Prochaska, J.O., & DiClemente, C.C. (1983). Stages and process of self-change of smoking: Toward an integrative model of change. *Journal of Consulting and Clinical Psychology*, **51**, 390-395.

Rahe, R.H., Ward, H.W., & Hayes,V. (1979). Brief group therapy in myocardial infarction rehabilitation: Three-to-four-year followup of a controlled trial. *Psychosomatic Medicine*, **41**, 229-242.

The Review Panel on Coronary-Prone Behavior and Coronary Heart Disease. (1981). Coronary-prone behavior and coronary heart disease: A critical review. *Circulation*, **63**, 1199-1215.

Rhoads, G.G. (1987). Reliability of diet measures as chronic disease risk factors. *American Journal of Clinical Nutrition*, **45**, 1073-1079.

Rogers, F., Juneau, M., Taylor, C.B., Haskell, N.L., Kraemer, H.C., Ahn, D.K., & DeBusk, R.F. (1987). Assessment by a microprocessor of adherence to home-based moderate intensity exercise training in healthy, sedentary middle-aged men and women. *American Journal of Cardiology*, **60**, 1-75.

Rosenman, R.H., Brand, R.J., Jenkins, C.D., Friedman, M., Straus, R., & Wurm, M. (1975). Coronary heart disease in the Western Collaborative Group

Study: Final follow-up experience of 8 1/2 years. *Journal of the American Medical Association*, **233**, 872-877.

Rossouw, J.E., Lewis, B., & Rifkind, B.M. (1990). The value of lowering cholesterol after myocardial infarction. *New England Journal of Medicine*, **323**, 1112-1119.

Ruberman, W., Weinblatt, E., Goldberg, J.D., & Chaudhary, B.S. (1984). Psychosocial influences on mortality after myocardial infarction. *New England Journal of Medicine*, **311**, 552-559.

Rudd, P. (1992). Maximizing compliance with antihypertensive therapy. *Drug Therapy*, **22**, 25-32.

Rudd, P., Ahmed, S., Zachary, V., Barton, C., & Bonduelle D. (1990). Improved compliance measures: Applications in an ambulatory hypertensive drug trial. *Clinical Pharmacology and Therapeutics*, **48**, 676-685.

Rudd, P., & Marshall, G. (1985). Antihypertensive medication taking behavior, outpatients patterns and implications. In J. Rosenfeld (Ed.), *Hypertensive control in the community* (pp. 232-236). London: John Libbey.

Sallis, J.F., Haskell, W.L., & Fortmann, S.P. (1986). Predictors of adoption and maintenance of physical activity in a community sample. *Preventive Medicine*, **15**, 331-341.

Sallis, J.F., Hill, J.D., Killen, J.D., Telch, M.J., Flora, J.A., Girard, J., & Taylor, C.B. (1986). Self-help smoking cessation compared to no treatment control. *American Journal of Preventive Medicine*, **2**, 342-344.

Schulberg, H.C., Saul, M., McClelland, M., Ganguli, M., Christy, W., & Frank, R. (1985). Assessing depression in primary medical and psychiatric practices. *Archives of General Psychiatry*, **42**, 1164-1170.

Shuster, J.L., Stern, T.A., & Tesar, G.E. (1992). Psychological problems and their management. In N.K. Wenger & H.K. Hellerstein (Eds.), *Rehabilitation of the Coronary Patient* (3rd ed., pp. 483-510). New York: Churchill Livingstone.

Sparrow, D., & Dawber, T.R. (1978). The influence of cigarette smoking on prognosis after a first myocardial infarction: A report from the Framingham Study. *Journal of Chronic Disorders*, **31**, 425-432.

Spielberger, C.D. (1983). *Manual of the State-Trait Anxiety Inventory (STAI Form Y)*. Palo Alto, CA: Consulting Psychologists Press.

Stern, M.J., & Cleary, P. (1981). National exercise and heart disease project: Psychosocial change observed during a low-level exercise program. *Archive of Internal Medicine*, **141**, 1463-1467.

Stubbe, I., Eskilsson, J., & Nilsson-Ehle, P. (1982). High-density lipoprotein concentrations increase after stopping smoking. *British Medical Journal of Clinical Research Education*, **284**, 1511-1513.

Taylor, C.B. (1987). Post-MI management. *Consultant*, **26**, 45-58.

Taylor, C.B., & Arnow, B. (1988). *The nature and treatment of anxiety disorders*. New York: Free Press.

Taylor, C.B., Bandura, A., Ewart, C.K., Miller, N.H., & DeBusk, R.F. (1985). Exercise testing to enhance wives' confidence in their husbands' cardiac capability soon after clinically uncomplicated myocardial infarction. *American Journal of Cardiology*, **55**, 635-638.

Taylor, C.B., DeBusk, R.F., Davidson, D.M., Houston, N., & Burnett, K. (1981). Optimal methods for identifying depression following hospitalization for myocardial infarction. *Journal of Chronic Diseases*, **34**, 127-133.

Taylor, C.B., Fortmann, S.P., Flora, J., Kayman, S., Barrett, D., Jatulis, D., & Farquhar, J.W. (1991). Effect of long-term community health education on body mass index: The Five-City Project. *American Journal of Epidemiology*, **134** (3), 235-249.

Taylor, C.B., & Houston Miller, N. (1989). Smoking cessation in patients with cardiovascular disease. *Quality of Life and Cardiovascular Care*, **5** (1), 19-35.

Taylor, C.B., & Houston Miller, N. (1993). Basic psychologic principles related to group exercise programs. In J.L. Durstine, A.C. King, & P. Painter (Eds.), *Resource manual for guidelines for exercise testing and prescription* (2nd ed., pp. 429-442). Philadelphia: Lea & Febiger.

Taylor, C.B., Houston Miller, N., Killen, J., & DeBusk, R.F. (1990). Smoking cessation after acute myocardial infarction: The effects of exercise training. *Addictive Behaviors*, **13**, 331-335.

Taylor, C.B., & Miller, N.H. (1992). Education and counseling of the patient and family: The behavioral approach. In N.K. Wenger & H.K. Hellerstein (Eds.), *Rehabilitation of the Coronary Patient* (pp. 461-471). New York: Churchill Livingstone.

Taylor, C.B., & Miller, N.H. (1993). Principles of health behavior change. In J.L. Durstine, A.C. King, P. Painter, et al. (Eds.), *Resource Manual for Guidelines for exercise Testing and Prescription* (2nd ed., pp. 429-535). Philadelphia: Lea & Febiger.

Taylor, C.B., Miller, N.H., Killen, J.D., & DeBusk, R.F. (1990). Smoking cessation after acute myocardial infarction: Effects of a nurse-managed intervention. *Annals of Internal Medicine*, **113**, 118-123.

Taylor, C.B., & Stunkard, A. (1993). Public health approaches to weight loss. In A.F. Stunkard & T.A. Wadden (Eds.), *Obesity: Theory and therapy* (pp. 335-353). New York: Raven Press.

Thomas, R.J., Miller, N.H., Lamendola-Rudd, C., Berra, K., Hedbäck, B., Durstine, J.L., & Haskell, W.L. (in press). Participation in cardiac rehabilitation programs by women and men: Results of a national survey.

Tonnesen, P., Fryd, V., Hansen, M., Helsted, J., Gunnersen, A.B., Forchammer, H., & Stockner, M. (1988). Effect of nicotine chewing gum in combination with group counseling on the cessation of smoking. *New England Journal of Medicine*, **318**, 15-18.

Transdermal Nicotine Study Group (1991). Transdermal nicotine for smoking cessation. *Journal of the American Medical Association*, **266**, 3133-3138.

U.S. Department of Health and Human Services. (1987). *The physician's guide: Improving adherence among hypertensive patients*.

Vinson, J.M., Rich, M.W., Sperry, J.C., Shah, A.S., & McNamara, T. (1990). Early re-admission of elderly patients with congestive heart failure. *Journal of American Geriatric Society*, **38**, 1290-1295.

Von Korff, M., Shapiro, S., Burke, J.D., Teitlebaum, M., Skinner, E.A., German, P., Turner, R.W., Klein, L., & Burns, B. (1987). Anxiety and depression in a primary care clinic: Comparison of Diagnostic Interview Schedule, General Health Questionnaire, and practitioner assessments. *Archives of General Psychiatry*, **44**, 152-156.

Wack, J.T., & Rodin, J. (1982). Smoking and its effects on body weight and systems of caloric regulation. *American Journal of Clinical Nutrition*, **35**, 366-380.

Wasson, J., Gaudette, C., Whaley, F., Sauvigne, A., Baribeau, P., & Welch, H.G. (1992). Telephone care as a substitute for routine clinic follow-up. *Journal of the American Medical Association*, **267**, 1788-1793.

Watson, D.L., & Tharp, R.G. (1981). *Self-directed behavior change*. Monterey: Brooks/Cole.

Watts, G.F., Lewis, B., Brunt, J.N., Lewis, E.S., Coltart, D.J., Smith, L.D., Mann, J.I., & Swan, A.V. (1992). Effects on coronary artery disease of lipid-lowering diet, or diet plus cholestyramine in the St. Thomas' Atherosclerosis Regression Study (STARS). *Lancet*, **339**, 563-569.

Wilhelmsson, C., Vedin, J.A., Elmfeldt, D., Tibblin, G., & Wilhelmsen, L. (1975). Smoking and myocardial infarction. *Lancet*, **1**, 415-420.

Williams, R.B., Barefoot, J.C., Califf, R.M., Haney, T.L., Saunders, W.B., Pryor, D.B., Hlatky, M.A., Siegler, I.C., & Mark, D.B. (1992). Prognostic importance of social and economic resources among medically treated patients with angiographically documented coronary artery disease. *Journal of the American Medical Association*, **267** (4), 520-524.

Williams, R.B., Haney, T., Lee, K.L., Kong, Y.H., Blumenthal, J.A., & Whalen, R.E. (1980). Type A behavior, hostility, and coronary heart disease. *Psychosomatic Medicine*, **42**, 539-549.

Winniford, M.D., Jansen, D.E., Reynolds, G.A., Apprill, P., Black, W.H., & Hillis, L.D. (1987). Cigarette smoking-induced coronary vasoconstriction in atherosclerotic coronary artery disease and prevention by calcium antagonists and nitroglycerin. *American Journal of Cardiology*, **59**, 203-207.

Wood, P.D., Stefanick, M.J., Williams, P.T., & Haskell, W.L. (1991). The effects on plasma lipoproteins of a prudent weight-reducing diet, with or without exercise in overweight men and women. *New England Journal of Medicine*, **325**, 461-466.

Zung, W.W.K. (1965). A self rating depression scale. *Archives of General Psychiatry*, **12**, 63-70.

Index

A

Abstinence Violation Effect, 13
Active Partnership™ program, 8, 81
  audiotapes, 81, 83, 88, 91-92, 94
  videotapes, 24, 53-54, 81, 82, 88, 93
  workbook, 23-24, 53, 81, 82-83, 88,
    90, 94
Adherence. *See* Exercise adherence and
    dropout; Medications, adherence to;
    Relapse, to smoking; Relapse pre-
    vention
Alcohol abuse
  anxiety and, 34
  helping patients with, 35-36
  incidence, 31, 32, 35
  referral guidelines, 35
  screening for, 32-33, 39
  smoking cessation and, 35, 92
  sources of information on, 35
American Heart Association, 4, 8
Anger, 31, 32, 38, 79-80
Anxiety
  alcohol abuse and, 34
  assessment of, 34
  description and causes, 34-35
  exercise adherence and, 49
  helping patients with, 26, 35
  history of SCRP research on, 2-3
  incidence, 31, 32, 34, 35
  referral guidelines, 35
  screening for, 31, 38
Assessment, of patients. *See also* Assess-
    ment, of progress; Screening, for
    psychosocial problems; Treadmill
    testing
  of dietary intake, 63-65, 69, 71, 73-75
  of exercise dropout potential, 49, 55
  exercise testing, 2, 51, 52, 53, 54
  for medication adherence, 106, 107,
    109-110
  of psychosocial problems, 33, 34, 36

  of readiness for change, 14
  for smoking cessation, 87-88, 89, 90-
    91, 96, 100-104
  of stress, 81, 82
Assessment, of programs, 22, 84, 86, 93
Assessment, of progress
  in dietary management, 69, 71
  in exercise training, 51, 52, 53, 54
  in stress management, 84
Audiotapes, Active Partnership™ series,
    81, 83, 88, 91-92, 94

B

Bandura, A., 3
Barbarowicz, Pat, 3-4
Beck Depression Inventory, 33
Behavior therapy theory, 11-12
Beta-blockers, and depression, 33
Block Questionnaires, The, 75

C

Caffeine, and stress, 82
CAGE Questionnaire, 32-33
CALS (Computer-Assisted Learning Sys-
    tem), 25, 71, 78
Cardiac rehabilitation programs. *See also*
    Stanford Cardiac Rehabilitation
    Program
  dropout from, 47, 49
  elements for success, 14-17
Cholesterol levels, lowering of, 1, 61, 66-
    67, 68, 71. *See also* Dietary manage-
    ment; HDL
Clark, Mia, 4
Cognitive factors. *See also* Education of
    patients
  in behavior therapy, 11-12
  social cognitive theory, 3, 7-11
Communication skills, 22-23
Computer-Assisted Learning System
    (CALS), 25, 71, 78
Computers, 25, 65, 71, 75, 78

Confidence. *See* Self-efficacy
Confrontation (communication technique)
  general principles, 23
  use for medication adherence, 109-110
  use with alcoholic patients, 36
Contracts and written agreements, 15-16,
    19, 50, 90
Cooking skills and cookbooks, 68, 77
Coronary Primary Prevention Trial
    (CPPT), 7

D

Daily exercise activity logs, 50-51, 53,
    54, 56
DeBusk, Robert F., 2
Depression
  anxiety and, 34
  assessment of, 33
  description and causes, 33
  exercise adherence and, 49
  helping patients with, 33-34
  history of SCRP research on, 2-3
  incidence, 31, 32, 33
  referral guidelines, 34
  screening for, 31, 38
Dietary management
  cardiovascular disease risk and, 61
  with co-morbid conditions, 69
  family support for, 20, 42, 45-46
  general considerations in, 62-63
  history of SCRP work with, 3
  intervention strategies, 65-71
  maintenance strategies, 70
  measuring intake for, 63-65, 69, 71,
    73-75
  MULTIFIT principles for, 17, 19-20
  recommendations summarized, 62
  referral guidelines, 69, 70
  for weight loss/management, 71-72
DietCoach™ program, 4
Diet Habit Survey, The, 75
Diet histories, 63
Dietitian's role, 61-62, 69, 70
Drop out, from exercise programs. *See*
    Exercise adherence and dropout

E

Education of patients. *See also* Printed
    materials for education; Videotapes
  assessment of programs for, 22

for exercise adherence, 53
general principles and methods, 21-25
history of SCRP work with, 3-4
for medication adherence, 105, 106-
    107, 108, 111-113
on smoking cessation, 87, 88, 89, 90,
    93, 94, 95, 97-99
in stress management, 81, 82-83
telephone follow-up and, 26
Efficacy. *See* Self-efficacy
Efficacy questionnaires, 67, 76, 90, 91,
    100
Evaluation, of patients. *See* Assessment,
    of patients; Assessment, of progress
Evaluation, of programs, 22, 84, 86, 93
Exercise. *See also* Exercise adherence
    and dropout; Exercise testing; Home
    exercise training
  cardiovascular disease risk and, 47
  psychological problems and, 34, 35
  self-monitoring of, 50-51, 53, 54, 56-
    58
  smoking cessation and, 47, 91
  for stress management, 47, 82
  for weight loss, 47, 72
Exercise adherence and dropout
  assessment of dropout potential, 49, 55
  dropout rates, 47
  factors in, 48-49
  family support and, 42, 46, 50, 51, 53
  with home exercise training, 48, 50,
    53-54
  intervention strategies, 50-53
  review of research on, 3, 4, 48, 53
Exercise Plan and Tip Sheet, 51, 59
Exercise testing, 2, 51, 52, 53, 54. *See
    also* Treadmill testing
Expectations, building accurate and posi-
    tive, 14-15, 19

F

Fagerström Tolerance Test of Nicotine
    Dependence, 89, 96
Family support. *See also* Social support;
    Spouses
  for dietary management, 20, 42, 45-46
  for exercise adherence, 42, 46, 50, 51,
    53
  for medication adherence, 106

MULTIFIT handout on, 37, 40-46
  for smoking cessation, 42, 46, 92
Feedback on patient progress (positive reinforcement)
  computerized, 25, 65, 71
  for dietary management, 20, 69, 71, 72
  for exercise adherence, 50, 51, 53, 54
  general principles, 16, 17
  in SCRP, 20, 25
  for smoking cessation, 93
Follow-up. *See also* Telephone follow-up
  for dietary management, 69-70
  for medication adherence, 29, 109-110
Food frequency assessment tools, 64-65, 71, 73-75
Food magazines, list of, 77
Food records, 63
Frequency, of food consumption
  for consumption of specific foods, 64-65, 71, 73-75
  of meals and snacks, 72

G

Generalization training, 52-53
Generalized Anxiety Disorder, 34
Goal setting, 15, 19, 50, 66-67, 70
Group intervention, 29-30, 36

H

Harvard-Willett Food Frequency Questionnaire, 75
Haskell, William L., 2
HDL (high-density lipoprotein), 85. *See also* Cholesterol levels, lowering of
Health Belief Model, 13-14
Health risk appraisal, computers for, 25
Heart rate monitors, 53, 54
High-density lipoprotein. *See* HDL
Home exercise training
  adherence to, 48, 50, 53-54
  SCRP use of, 2, 26-27
  social support and, 50
  telephone monitoring of, 26-27, 28
Hostility, in cardiovascular disease risk, 79-80. *See also* Anger
Hyperlipidemic Diet Intervention for MULTIFIT, 19-20

I

Information for patients. *See* Education of patients; Printed materials for education; Videotapes

Information for Spouses, 37, 40-46
Interpersonal communication, 22-23
Ischemic heart disease, and smoking, 85, 86

K

Kaiser Permanente Medical Centers, 4, 32-33

L

Listening skills, 23
Logs, of exercise activity, 50-51, 53, 54, 56-58

M

Magazines on food, list of, 77
Marlatt's relapse prevention model, 12-13
Medication Information Sheet, 106, 107, 111-113
Medications, adherence to
  assessment of patients for, 106, 107, 109-110
  factors in, 105, 110
  follow-up/monitoring of, 29, 108, 109-110
  intervention strategies, 105-109
  self-efficacy and, 11, 12
  statistics on, 105, 109
Monitoring. *See* Follow-up; Self-monitoring; Telephone follow-up
Monthly exercise activity logs, 53
Morbidity. *See* Mortality and morbidity
Mortality and morbidity
  alcohol abuse and, 35
  depression and, 33
  exercise and, 47
  inadequate social support and, 36
  smoking and, 85, 86
  stress and, 79, 80
Motivation. *See* Exercise adherence and dropout
Multifactorial Risk Factor Intervention Trial (MRFIT), 7
MULTIFIT Daily Exercise Log, 50-51, 53, 54, 56
MULTIFIT Information for Spouses, 37, 40-46
MULTIFIT program
  for dietary management, 17, 19-20, 65, 71, 73-74
  for exercise training, 50-51, 53-54, 56-58

MULTIFIT program (*continued*)
  general intervention methods in, 23-25
  history of, 4
  for medication adherence, 106-108
  psychological screening in, 31-33, 38-39
  relapse prevention model in, 13
  self-efficacy assessment in, 10-11, 12
  for smoking cessation, 87, 88, 91-92, 93-94
  spousal support in, 37, 40-46
  stress management in, 81-84

N

National Clearinghouse for Alcohol and Drug Information, 35
National Heart, Lung, and Blood Institute (NHLBI), 4
Nicotine Chewing Gum Patient Information, 89, 97-98
Nicotine Transderm Patch Patient Information, 90, 99
Nicotine withdrawal. *See also* Smoking; Smoking cessation
  addiction assessment and, 89, 96
  low-nicotine cigarette smoking for, 86-87
  nicotine replacement therapy for, 89-90, 93-94, 97-99
Nutrition improvement. *See* Dietary management

O

Obesity, exercise adherence and, 49. *See also* Weight loss; Weight management
Outcome measures, for programs, 22, 84, 86, 93. *See also* Assessment, of progress

P

Panic Disorder, 34
Patient education. *See* Education of patients
PepsiCo Foundation, 3
Physician Advice Statement for Smoking, 87, 95
Positive reinforcement. *See* Feedback on patient progress; Rewards
Pre-Exercise Assessment Questionnaire, 49, 55

Printed materials for education
  for dietary management, 68, 77
  for exercise adherence, 53
  on family support issues, 37, 40-46
  guidelines for developing, 23-24
  for smoking cessation, 87, 88, 89, 90, 94, 95, 97-99
  for stress management, 81, 82-83
Problem solving
  in dietary management, 20, 67
  general principles, 16
  in medication adherence, 106, 109
  in stress management, 83
Program assessment, 22, 84, 86, 93
Progress assessment. *See* Assessment, of progress
Prompts, 16, 20, 107-108
Psychological aspects of recovery. *See also* Anger; Anxiety; Depression; Stress, management of; Stress, problems with
  history of SCRP research on, 2-3
  referral guidelines, 34, 35
  screening for problems with, 31-33, 38-39, 82
Psychosocial Questionnaire, 31-33, 38-39, 82

Q

Quantitative Food Frequency Analysis, The, 75

R

Readiness for change, 14
Readiness for learning, 22
Referral
  for alcohol problems, 35
  for dietary management, 69, 70
  for psychological problems, 34, 35
  for smoking cessation, 88, 90
  for social support problems, 36
  for stress management, 84
Relapse, to smoking, 35, 85-86, 91, 92, 94. *See also* Exercise adherence and dropout; Relapse prevention
Relapse prevention
  for dietary management, 19, 70
  for exercise adherence, 51-52
  general principles, 16
  history of SCRP work with, 3, 19

Marlatt's model for, 12-13
  for medication adherence, 108
  for smoking cessation, 3, 26, 47, 90-93
  stress management for, 80
Relaxation procedures, 81, 82, 83, 91-92
Responsibility issues, 17-18
Rewards, 17, 20. *See also* Feedback on
    patient progress
Role modeling, 8, 16, 19, 68

S
Screening, for psychosocial problems, 31-
    33, 38-39, 82
SCRP. *See* Stanford Cardiac Rehabilita-
    tion Program
Self-efficacy
  dietary management and, 67, 71, 76
  history of SCRP research on, 2-3, 9-11,
    12
  medication adherence and, 11, 12
  smoking cessation and, 88, 90, 91, 100
  theory of, 8, 9
Self-efficacy questionnaires, 67, 76, 90,
    91, 100
Self-monitoring
  of dietary management, 72
  of exercise, 50-51, 53, 54, 56-58
  of medication adherence, 108
  of stress, 81
Self-testing, for exercise progress assess-
    ment, 51, 52, 53
Side effects of medication
  depression, 33
  medication adherence and, 105, 107,
    108-109
  of nicotine replacement therapy, 89,
    90, 97-98, 99
Smoking
  in cardiovascular disease risk, 85
  exercise adherence and, 49
  stress and, 82
Smoking cessation
  alcohol abuse and, 35, 92
  assessment of patients, 87-88, 89, 90-
    91, 96, 100-104
  assessment of programs, 86, 93
  cardiovascular disease risk and, 1, 85
  exercise and, 47, 91
  family support for, 42, 46, 92

history of SCRP work with, 3, 4
  intervention strategies, 86-94
  referral guidelines, 88, 90
  relapse from, 35, 85-86, 91, 92, 94
  relapse prevention, 3, 26, 47, 90-93
  stress management and, 82, 91-92
  telephone follow-up for, 26, 28, 93, 94,
    101-104
  weight management and, 92-93
Social cognitive theory, 3, 7-11
Social support. *See also* Family support;
    Spouses
  for dietary management, 20
  for exercise adherence, 49, 50, 51
  general principles, 17
  group interventions for, 29-30, 36
  inadequate, 32, 36-37, 39
  for smoking cessation, 92
  telephone follow-up for, 30, 36, 37, 50
Spouses. *See also* Family support; Social
    support
  exercise adherence and, 50, 51
  informational handout for, 37, 40-46
  rehabilitation program success in gen-
    eral and, 17
  self-efficacy judgments of, 9-10
  smoking cessation and, 92
Stanford Cardiac Rehabilitation Program
    (SCRP). *See also* MULTIFIT
    program
  Computer-Assisted Learning System
    (CALS), 25, 71, 78
  feedback in, 20, 25
  history of, 1-5
  self-efficacy research by, 2-3, 9-11, 12
Stanford Five-Cities Project, 4, 7
"Staying Cool" (stress management man-
    ual), 81
Stress, management of
  assessment of programs for, 84
  cardiovascular disease risk and, 79-80
  exercise for, 47, 82
  history of SCRP research on, 4
  intervention techniques, 36, 81-84
  outcome measurement, 84
  referral guidelines, 84
  for relapse prevention, 80
  smoking cessation and, 82, 91-92
  theoretical models for, 81

Stress, problems with
  assessment of, 81, 82
  incidence, 32
    reening for, 31, 38

T

TABP (Type A Behavior Pattern), 79-80
Telephone follow-up
  for dietary management, 69-70
  for exercise adherence, 50, 53, 54
  guidelines for, 27-29
  history of SCRP use of, 2
  problems with, 28-29
  psychological problems and, 26
  review of research on, 26-27, 28, 29
  for smoking cessation, 26, 28, 93, 94,
    101-104
  for social support, 30, 36, 37, 50
  for stress management/monitoring, 36,
    81, 82, 83-84
Telephone Interview for Patients At-
    tempting to Quit Smoking, 93, 101-
    104
Theory
  of behavior therapy, 11-12
  Health Belief Model, 13-14
  on readiness to change, 14
  relapse prevention model, 12-13

  social cognitive, 3, 7-11
Treadmill testing
  for feedback on progress, 51, 52, 53,
    54
  physical effects of, 2
  self-efficacy and, 9
Twenty-four hour recall (dietary intake as-
    sessment tool), 64
Type A Behavior Pattern (TABP), 79-80

V

Videotapes
  effectiveness of, 24-25
  for exercise adherence, 53-54
  for role modeling, 16, 19
  for smoking cessation, 88, 93
  for stress management, 81, 82

W

Weekly Exercise Activity Log, 51, 54, 58
Weight loss, 4, 47, 61, 71-72. *See also*
    Dietary management
Weight management, 49, 71-72, 92
    See also Dietary management;
    Weight loss
Written agreements/contracts, 15-16, 19,
    50, 90

About the Authors

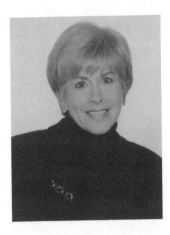

Nancy Houston Miller

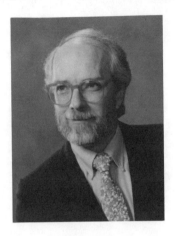

Craig Barr Taylor

Nancy Houston Miller is the associate director of the nationally recognized Stanford Cardiac Rehabilitation Program. Having worked in cardiac rehabilitation for more than 20 years, she has a thorough understanding of what it takes to help patients with coronary heart disease change their lifestyles. Her extensive research in cardiovascular risk reduction has involved work on the development of MULTIFIT, the multiple risk factor intervention program described in this monograph. Since 1973 she has worked with patients in the YMCArdiac Therapy Exercise Program, now known as the Cardiac Therapy Foundation of the Mid-Peninsula, in Palo Alto, CA.

A member of both the American Association of Cardiovascular and Pulmonary Rehabilitation and the American Heart Association, Houston Miller received fellowship awards from these organizations in 1990 and 1991, respectively. She earned her bachelor's degree in nursing from the University of Washington in 1972.

Craig Barr Taylor is the codirector of the Stanford Cardiac Rehabilitation Program. A board-certified psychiatrist, he has more than two decades of experience in clinical and research interventions with coronary heart disease patients. He has been a professor of psychiatry at Stanford University School of Medicine since 1991.

Taylor was a principal investigator on the MULTIFIT research study, a project funded by the National Heart, Lung, and Blood Institute. He, Houston Miller, and others are responsible for developing the American Heart Association's Active Partnership™ Program, which has been used with more than one million patients. A member of the American Association of Cardiopulmonary Rehabilitation and the Society of Behavioral Medicine, Taylor was elected president of the latter organization for the 1995 term. He earned his MD in 1970 from the University of Utah College of Medicine.

More great books for cardiac rehab specialists

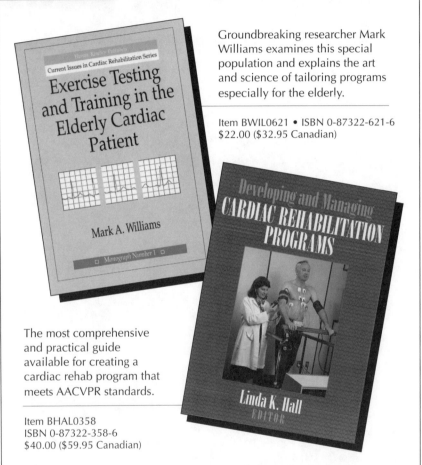

Groundbreaking researcher Mark Williams examines this special population and explains the art and science of tailoring programs especially for the elderly.

Item BWIL0621 • ISBN 0-87322-621-6
$22.00 ($32.95 Canadian)

The most comprehensive and practical guide available for creating a cardiac rehab program that meets AACVPR standards.

Item BHAL0358
ISBN 0-87322-358-6
$40.00 ($59.95 Canadian)

To place an order: U.S. customers call **TOLL-FREE 1-800-747-4457**.
Customers outside of U.S. use the appropriate telephone
number/address shown in the front of this book.

HUMAN KINETICS
The Information Leader in Physical Activity
P.O. Box 5076, Champaign, IL 61825-5076
www.humankinetics.com

Prices subject to change.